Posthumanism and Public Health

The intellectual and moral imperatives that underscore public health have sustained the idea that its fundamental scope is the study of human health, illness and suffering, and that these are self-evidently attributable to individuals and groups of people. This edited collection explores to what extent a shift towards more posthuman perspectives – where the status of the human as the obvious focus for our attention is de-stabilised – might catalyse complimentary or alternative accounts of common topics in public health. The collection argues that through this posthuman approach, standard categories such as health, illness and even the body might be re-conceived as interactions between people, other living things, material objects and the environment – rather than as inherently human properties.

By taking into greater account the relationships between humans and non-humans, this approach re-casts many of the traditional topics in public health, and offers new opportunities for examining them. In so doing, the book raises key questions about researching 'health'; about considering the extent to which it may be productive to think about public health beyond the interests of human lives; and what happens to our moral and ethical commitments if we no longer put humans first.

This book was originally published as a special issue of *Critical Public Health*.

Simon Cohn is Professor in Medical Anthropology at the London School of Hygiene & Tropical Medicine, UK. Drawing increasingly on science studies and practice theory, his research has focused on issues related to diagnosis, contested conditions and chronic illness in the UK and other high-income societies.

Rebecca Lynch is a Research Fellow in Medical Anthropology at the London School of Hygiene & Tropical Medicine, UK. Her research is interested in constructions of the body, health and illness particularly in relation to morality, values and categorisation. She has undertaken ethnographic fieldwork in Trinidad and research projects in the UK.

Posthumanism and Public Health

Edited by
Simon Cohn and Rebecca Lynch

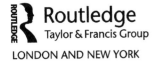

LONDON AND NEW YORK

First published 2018 by Routledge

2 Park Square, Milton Park, Abingdon, Oxfordshire OX14 4RN
52 Vanderbilt Avenue, New York, NY 10017

Routledge is an imprint of the Taylor & Francis Group, an informa business

First issued in paperback 2019

British Library Cataloguing in Publication Data
A catalogue record for this book is available from the British Library

ISBN 13: 978-1-138-10457-0 (hbk)
ISBN 13: 978-0-367-26487-1 (pbk)

Typeset in Myriad Pro
by RefineCatch Limited, Bungay, Suffolk

Publisher's Note
The publisher accepts responsibility for any inconsistencies that may have
arisen during the conversion of this book from journal articles to book chapters,
namely the possible inclusion of journal terminology.

Disclaimer
Every effort has been made to contact copyright holders for their permission to
reprint material in this book. The publishers would be grateful to hear from any
copyright holder who is not here acknowledged and will undertake to rectify
any errors or omissions in future editions of this book.

Contents

Citation Information

The chapters in this book were originally published in *Critical Public Health*, volume 27, no. 3 (June 2017). When citing this material, please use the original page numbering for each article, as follows:

Editorial
Posthuman perspectives: relevance for a global public health
Simon Cohn and Rebecca Lynch
Critical Public Health, volume 27, no. 3 (June 2017), pp. 285–292

Chapter 1
On difference and doubt as tools for critical engagement with public health
Catherine M. Will
Critical Public Health, volume 27, no. 3 (June 2017), pp. 293–302

Chapter 2
Posthumanist critique and human health: how nonhumans (could) figure in public health research
Carrie Friese and Nathalie Nuyts
Critical Public Health, volume 27, no. 3 (June 2017), pp. 303–313

Chapter 3
Who or what is 'the public' in critical public health? Reflections on posthumanism and anthropological engagements with One Health
Melanie J. Rock
Critical Public Health, volume 27, no. 3 (June 2017), pp. 314–324

Chapter 4
Enacting toxicity: epidemiology and the study of air pollution for public health
Emma Garnett
Critical Public Health, volume 27, no. 3 (June 2017), pp. 325–336

Chapter 5
The injecting 'event': harm reduction beyond the human
Fay Dennis
Critical Public Health, volume 27, no. 3 (June 2017), pp. 337–349

For any permission-related enquiries please visit:
http://www.tandfonline.com/page/help/permissions

Notes on Contributors

Simon Cohn, Department of Health Services Research & Policy, London School of Hygiene & Tropical Medicine, London, UK.

Fay Dennis, Department of Sociology, Goldsmiths, University of London, London, UK.

Carrie Friese, Sociology Department, London School of Economics and Political Science, London, UK.

Emma Garnett, Health Services Research & Policy, London School of Hygiene & Tropical Medicine, London, UK.

Dominique Grimard, Institute of Public Health Research of University of Montreal (IRSPUM), Montreal, Canada.

Pascale Lehoux, Department of Health Management, Evaluation and Policy, University of Montreal; Institute of Public Health Research of University of Montreal (IRSPUM), University of Montreal; Research Chair on Responsible Innovation in Health, Montreal, Canada.

Rebecca Lynch, Department of Health Services Research & Policy, London School of Hygiene & Tropical Medicine, London, UK.

Elizabeth Mills, Department of Anthropology, University of Sussex, Brighton, UK.

Nathalie Nuyts, Sociology Department, London School of Economics and Political Science, London, UK.

Sébastien Proulx, Institute of Public Health Research of University of Montreal (IRSPUM), Montreal, Canada.

Melanie J. Rock, Department of Community Health Sciences, Cumming School of Medicine, University of Calgary, Canada; Department of Ecosystem and Public Health, Faculty of Veterinary Medicine, University of Calgary, Canada; O'Brien Institute for Public Health, University of Calgary, Canada.

Mette N. Svendsen, Department of Public Health, Centre for Medical Science and Technology Studies, University of Copenhagen, Copenhagen, Denmark.

Catherine M. Will, School of Law, Politics and Sociology, Freeman Centre, University of Sussex, Brighton, UK.

B. Williams-Jones, Department of Social and Preventive Medicine, University of Montreal, Institute of Public Health Research of University of Montreal (IRSPUM), Montreal, Canada.

Posthuman perspectives: relevance for a global public health

In this special issue of *Critical Public Health* the papers collectively explore how certain theoretical perspectives in the social sciences, often termed 'posthumanism', might productively be applied to public health research. In this introduction we want to argue that this is much more than an academic exercise that simply follows intellectual fashion, to show its value for those engaged in a wide range of research and applied work. More than this, we also want to argue how it has the potential to reinvigorate a key argument that some readers may fear is disappearing from view – that talking about health is talking about politics.

From the outset, however, we need to acknowledge that the perspectives we are referring to are resolutely heterogeneous. Whilst there are some who have attempted to define and delimit what posthumanism might mean (see Braidotti, 2015; Wolfe, 2010), many of the theorists our contributors draw on might either reject the label, or feel they have little in common with other writers they are associated with. Nevertheless, it is at least possible to make clear what posthumanism does not refer to, and state a few common features.

First, it is important to emphasise that in all of the papers in this special issue there is no attempt to link posthumanism to *transhumanism*. This latter term refers to ways in which the current capacities of human beings might be enhanced by technology in order to go beyond what we take to be our normal biological potential (Bostrom, 2005). Transhumanism therefore engages with ideas of non-organic, biological and pharmaceutical enhancement. But while some of this literature cautions on the ethical consequences of making humans more than they currently are (McNamee & Edwards, 2006), much of this work has a celebratory, science-fiction orientation, not to say messianic sentiment, given that forms of transhumanism have morphed into a number of new religious movements (e.g. see Tirosh-Samuelson, 2012). Although there is apparent cross over between this literature and certain terms adopted by posthuman theorists who talk of the cyborg (Haraway, 1991) or hybrid (Latour, 2005), they do so mainly to invoke processes of melding, mixing and the unsettling existing categories, rather than as literal accounts of human augmentation.

We would argue that drawing on posthuman perspectives offers much more than merely a concern for new possibilities for human existence. Rather, it reflects an interest across many academic disciplines – including geography, sociology, anthropology, science and technology studies, and feminism – to reframe current social enquiry by looking more carefully at the role non-human elements, such as objects, other organisms and the environment play. At one level this is far from new. For example, all readers will of course know the iconic story of John Snow and the Broad Street pump handle. Notwithstanding evidence that suggests the removal of the pump handle was perhaps not as significant as originally claimed (Krieger, 1992), it nevertheless continues to be represented as having been central to stemming the outbreak of cholera in Soho, London in the mid-nineteenth century. But a more contemporary, posthuman account might well say the bar of iron constituted a significant *actor*. What is the point of telling the story this way, and risking the wrath of critics who dismiss the use of words such as 'actor' and 'agency' to non-human elements? (See Elder-Vass, 2015; for just such a retaliation.) At one level, the point is simple; to present accounts of humans and non-humans in common ways, so that we don't inadvertently assume from the outset that one is more important, or has more influence, than any other. In other words, if we are going to present the impoverished Soho dwellers as actors, then why not also the handle which was just as important – since only in combination could the contaminated water be obtained? This point illustrates a posthumanism conviction not to automatically accord humans with an exceptional status, and instead find ways to present non-human elements with equivalence. This is what some people mean when they talk about adopting a 'flat ontology' (Law, 2004). The result is that we should not assume from the outset that humans will always be the central focus of our attention, but they instead constitute only one category amongst a range of different kinds of actors.

Now, it is clear that by introducing the theme of this special issue in this way it may well appear to be an unlikely topic for the CPH readership, given we are all centrally committed to research and debate that might influence the health and lives of people, and tend to include other things only so far as they might causally impact on humans. So first, let us offer two levels of response that, in combination, suggest how broadening a focus beyond humans to take non-humans seriously might have genuine value.

The value of reframing

Our first response to the question of what posthumanism might offer public health concerns its critical potential. All the papers in this issue demonstrate, in different ways, how one can draw judiciously from this body of theoretical work to re-imagine and re-problematise public health topics by both foregrounding things not normally attended to and by questioning those that might be taken for granted. This directly engages with one aspect of any critical enquiry – the imperative to find ways to conceive of issues in radically new ways, so that different aspects might fall under scrutiny.

To illustrate this, let us start with a brief anecdote. At a conference we both went to recently a number of senior academics, reacting against some of the presentations inspired by these new theoretical debates, in unison retorted, 'It's ludicrous. Forests can't think!' They were referring to an ethnography that has become synonymous with posthuman trends, in which the anthropologist, Kohn, describes how the Runa, an indigenous peoples of Amazonia, understand all living things to be part of a single biological complex that is able to perceive, process and respond (Kohn, 2013). But Kohn goes further than anthropologists might usually do. Rather than merely present this as a cultural representation that can be explained away as a 'local belief', he explores ways in which Runa ideas about thinking might legitimately be attributed to ecological systems. The error of those senior academics, then, was their failure to recognise that considering the possibility a nonhuman entity can think is an important, if playful, provocation to ask what thinking 'is', and to what extent usual definitions implicitly reproduce cultural, anthropocentric, assumptions. Attributing something such as thought to the nonhuman does not merely reveal how an apparently neutral concept articulates particular values, but in the process of seeing how it might be attributed to a non-human entity – in this case a rainforest – that it can radically unsettle and reinvigorate how we approach the topic.

Of course, Kohn is in no way the first to do this when it comes to the question of thought. One could justifiably claim that Turing explored the same thing in his well-known experiment to test machine-based artificial intelligence (1950). As Turing himself noted, the test is not designed to assess whether machines can think like humans, but whether humans might be led to reason that machines think like them. What is productive in both these instances – one concerning the natural environment and the other technology – is the inherent looping between applying terms and ideas to new entities and contexts, and then recognising the extent to which they might have to be reformulated or resisted. Although this continual fluidity may well be frustrating, especially for positivists, it can nevertheless have enormous scholarly value because it forces us to continually question not 'how things are,' but 'what version of how things are should we adopt, and why?' Here, then, in the productive potential of reframing already lies some of the political potential of a posthuman approach.

Health as relational

So far, we have implicitly explored the question of the utility of posthuman perspectives for public health in terms of general methodology – the nature of data that might be collected, and how best to deploy analytical categories in order to incorporate that data into our accounts. A stronger response does not reject these points, but argues matters relating to human health and illness can never be simply divided from their entanglements with nonhuman things, and that to demarcate them off dramatically limits where and how we might intervene.

It is a truism to say that the intellectual and moral commitments underscoring public health are driven by the fundamental aim of studying and improving human health. However, in different contexts the idea of 'health' is regularly applied to other things as well; we talk about animal health, plant health, the health of the environment, and even now the health of the internet. What is of note is that in all these cases the health in question is usually defined and assessed according to entity-specific criteria. But the potential of a posthuman approach, which emphases putting non-human elements as level actors alongside humans, is that the category of health might itself might have to be broadened and re-conceived as generalised and shared. Rather than a property of a body or entity, the meaning shifts to being a quality of relationships between humans, other living things, the environment and even material objects.

This, too, if far from a new point to make; public health has long emphasised a more relational approach to health research. But traditionally, many of the so-called 'biopsychosocial environmental' models, especially those derived from epidemiology, nevertheless place the human at the centre of various domains of influence (e.g. Engel, 1977). In contrast, a posthuman perspective attempts to dissolve the human centrality by recognising relationships are dispersed and distributed, leading to a conceptualisation of health as a diffuse quality across diverse entities that include the human, but cannot be attributed solely to the human. Accepting this suggests not only that 'human health' is always co-produced though the nature of interactions and relations with non-humans, but that delineating human from non-human health might foreclose theoretical insight and practical potential.

Beyond the call to adopt a much broader, flatter, perspective, posthuman approaches also tend to resist describing the relationships between things as a system or bounded field. The argument is that such models and representations are only ever artefacts of the researcher who seeks tidy explanations and accounts. In so doing, inherent mess and constant transformation is substituted for order and enclosure. The alternative is to emphasise the ephemeral and context-specific nature of various assemblages of things (see for e.g. Jensen & Winthereik, 2013). What might be said to be the case in one context is unlikely to be so in another, as each historical and geographic circumstance shapes what things are brought together and how they relate. However, this is not intended to be an argument for extreme relativism; rather, the emphasis is put on us – as researchers, readers and practitioners – to think more carefully about what aspects of any findings or insights might be relevant elsewhere, and what are rooted to the specific. In this way, not only does the focus of health research shift from the human to being a more distributed quality across heterogeneous relationships, but the analytical approach must resist trying to encompass everything into a single neat, causally ordered account.

The human focus of public health

As we have discussed, despite different disciplinary approaches and foci, public health champions a concern with human health at a collective level. But in addition to potentially reconfiguring what the boundaries of health might legitimately constitute, the very category of what it is to be human is also worth interrogating. Clearly, the question of what it is to be human has been central to Western thought for millennia. Arguably, our contemporary ideas are most influenced by writing from the Enlightenment on human nature, human rights and human reason (Morris, 1991; Redfield, 2013), which themselves drew on texts from the Renaissance and Ancient Greeks. Being an era of optimism, triumph, new wealth and conquest (for some) shaped the proliferation of treaties on essential and universal human qualities such as autonomy, stability, freedom, rationality, free-will, integrity and so on. Accordingly, these characteristics provided the reasoning behind further key distinctions, such as mind/body, culture/nature, animal/human, living/dead. We would argue that these qualities and distinctions continue to be articulated in much of the contemporary work of public health; from its laudable concern with health inequalities, differential access to health care, and the political economy of health generally, the commitment to fairness and justice are based on deep-rooted ideas about human potential and dignity. They are also very present in much of the rise of global health, as a revision of earlier development and aid discourses. Many advocates argue that at its core global health should concern the worldwide delivery approaches to human distress and suffering through a language of universal human rights and ethics (Koplan et al., 2009). But these refined and abstract ideas associated with the human are never neutral. The same historical drives that led to essential claims emphasising the discrete, exceptional status of the human (Carrithers, Collins, & Lukes, 1985) also ensured that the default human was white, male, adult and privileged (Oudshoorn, 2003). These normative qualities were consequently borne from privilege and power. The central point is that even an entity that may appear innocuous and common sense – that of the human – is not merely a cultural, but also a political category.

Despite the dominance of this representation, both historical events and theoretical writings during in the late nineteenth century increasingly unsettled confidence in what it is to be human. For example, the so called three-member 'party of suspicion' coined by Ricoeur (see Scott-Baumann, 2009), referring to Marx, Nietzsche and Freud, in combination emphasised how humans were not as noble, rational, aware or controlled as we might have wanted to believe. And later, during the twentieth century, further de-stabilisation from such domains as feminism, gender politics, critical race theory, identity studies and queer theory emphasised the inherent patriarchal nature of 'the human'. In response, they suggested subverting ideas of integrity, continuity and rationality with a new language of fragmentation, multiplicity, instability, play and hybridity. More recently, a different body of knowledge has contributed to this unsettling; that of biology itself. Scholars have drawn on this to think about the permeability of skin (Diamond, 2013), the vast numbers of bacterial cells in the human gut (Landecker, 2016), and the never-ending difficulty in deciding when human life begins and ends (Helmreich, 2015) in order to highlight how any representation of what it is to be human inescapably enlists non-scientific values and criteria as well as scientific categories and definitions.

Crucially, one of the qualities of a posthuman approach in response to all these challenges is not to seek to resolve such ambiguity, or adopt a working definition for pragmatic purposes, but instead to accept and exploit ambivalence in order to highlight those values. One can see the legacy of these earlier debates in a variety of posthumanist subject areas: the environment, ecosystems and debates about nature; discussions about technology, information and data; human-animal relations, and the one-health agenda; material culture and new materialism; bacteria, the microbiome and anti-microbial resistance. Within all of these, a key notion of the 'human' is replaced with approaches that recognise the contingent and co-constituted nature of humans as they exist through multiple relationships with other things. Such posthuman perspectives are not driven by a desire for academic novelty, but from the fact that the old category increasingly does not work, or make sense, when one attends to the multiple relationships between what are traditionally thought of as human and nonhuman materialities and concerns.

At this stage of discussion we arrive at new questions. What do we retain that is inherently 'public health' if we are open to revise both what 'public' and 'health' can refer to? And how might posthumanism be drawn on to do politics? Politics has never been so in the forefront of our minds. And yet, in this so-called post-fact, post-party world, it is not always straightforward to work out how one should articulate a political position.

Decades ago, the stalwart critical thinker Habermas had a very public quarrel with the social theorist Lyotard on the complacent conservatism of postmodernism (Habermas & Levin, 1982). Habermas not only pointed to the apparent extreme relativism of postmodern thought that potentially undermined any means to take a stand, but charged many theorists with indulgent self-referential playfulness for its own sake. One way of understanding this dispute is not in terms of political conviction, but rather in terms of what the project of academic research might actually be. For Habermas and many who follow a traditional Marxist line of thinking, the central purpose is to catalyse emancipation through forms of 'unmasking' (Rorty, 1984). However, what authors such as Lyotard, Deleuze, Foucault and Baudrillard were moving to was not a total rejection of Marxism, but a worry that any project of unmasking implied one can be certain about how things really are beneath. As an alternative, they therefore shifted from the project of unmasking to a focus on the work of signs, representations, discourses and metanarratives. Rather than considering these to be modes of concealment, they were conceived to be ways in which power is articulated through constructions of reality.

Posthumanism could be said to have adopted much from this strategy. Given relationships between humans and non-humans are infinite, and that the category of the human is itself a result of these relationships rather than essential biological or moral characteristics, it only ever offers a partial representation to invite re-evaluation and appraisal, rather than definitive claims of truth. So politics no longer is about identifying certainties, or defending absolutes, but rather about opening up new spaces and relationships for engagement. This may well seem like a much weaker and timid politics to that of Marxist totality (Jay, 1984). But one might say as a response, it nevertheless provides a subtle kind of politics, that is perhaps more apt and productive in our current times.

The collection

In this introduction we have argued that adopting a posthumanist perspective has the capacity to reconfigure existing concerns, and open up radically new lines of enquiry. Posthumanism is thus an intellectual exercise that should be taken seriously because it has the potential not only to generate productive and practical alternative accounts, but because it may well identify new spaces and opportunities to intervene. Thus, posthuman perspectives are not about leaving what is human behind, but in fact the opposite – exploring what being human means in relation to what might be deemed as not human.

This special issue therefore explores new configurations that attend to the mutual relationships between people, other living things, objects and environments in order to illustrate how, by attending to these, traditional public health topics might be recast. Ethnographic approaches appear particularly useful for this endeavour, given their commitment not to pursue an a priori hypothesis and their requirement for reflexive engagement. As a discipline at home with such methods, six of the contributors are unsurprisingly therefore anthropologists who have conducted in-depth fieldwork that takes the non-human as a key part of their ethnographic focus. Their papers reflect this methodological challenge to more open-ended, if not experimental, in order to incorporate those things not normally considered central. And more generally across the papers in the issue, diverse sources of data – such as body mapping, photography and film, as well as scatter plot graphs, co-citation analysis and a futuristic thought experiment – further demonstrate the quest to escape standard approaches to research and explore a topic.

We start the collection with an engagement with the past, juxtaposing established and familiar sociological perspectives with posthuman theorists. This first paper provides a theoretical review that contextualizes the potential of posthumanism to provide new tools for public health enquiry. Making links between contrasting approaches, Will (2017) holds a 'conversation' between Foucault and posthuman scholars, suggesting that the latter provide space to acknowledge multiplicity and attend to public health practices of care. Will proposes that such reframing draws attention to inequalities and to the entangled relationships between humans and non-humans. This overview is further developed in Friese and Nuyts (2017) analysis of the growth of public health research involving non-humans. Paying particular attention to writing on animals the authors identify a place to extend debate further, and identify the One Health movement as a partial precursor to posthuman approaches; partial because, although it sees population health as a combination of human and animal health, it does not go far enough. But by rigorously 'following the non-humans' the authors suggest public health could both benefit from, and contribute to, an emerging field. These first two papers therefore contextualise and set posthuman debates within existing theory and developing areas of interest in public health, identifying key spaces in which posthumanism has the potential to contribute. How such approaches are drawn on in the gathering, analysis and framing of research undertaken within public health are then taken up in the other papers in the collection.

In order to attend to the non-human in their work, the majority of the remaining contributions capture many of those aspects of research that might normally be considered 'background'. In the first of these, Rock takes up the specific theme of human-animal relations brought to the fore by Friese and Nuyts through a study of dog walking in Canada. Rock (2017) draws on contemporary anthropological work that strives to examine the intimate and often mutually beneficial relationship between people and animals. The author uses this to then ask what 'the public' in public health might look like if we incorporate non-humans, and to what extent might our understandings of public health change. Implicit in her argument is a political question about voice and representation; who is able to speak, and who is able to speak for whom? While Rock questions the notion of the 'public', Garnett (2017) goes on to question our understanding of 'health'. Based on her participatory fieldwork with epidemiologists studying air pollution, Garnett's work draws out changing constructions of health from within science as epidemiologists try to pin down a notion of 'health' which makes sense of their heterogeneous, and sometimes apparently contradictory, data. Through a variety of creative techniques, in which researchers try to establish relations between air pollution and epidemiological data, 'health' becomes configured beyond the human as a distributed and relational phenomenon that takes into account ideas of space, volume and the changing of seasons. In both Garnett's and Rock's work a central concern is how aspects of the environment not only impact on human health and wellbeing but can be seen to constitute it.

Taking a different but related move, the next three papers explicitly examine how material technologies extend into human bodies themselves, reframing how bodies are constructed, how they can be seen as joined to each other and wider socio-cultural dynamics, and how bodily substances are transformed through materials and practices. All three adopt a dynamic description the body and to human-nonhuman relations, accentuating movement, flow and transformation in the intermingling of the human and nonhuman. In the first of these, Dennis (2017) takes a posthuman approach to drug-taking in order to critically explore current techniques of harm reduction. She argues that most of these implicitly construct a rationalist drug user as the focus of medical intervention, but ignore the relationality between bodies, words, substances and things that form collective participation in what she terms 'the injecting event'. Dennis uses body maps not to record a final representation of how drug users view themselves, but rather as a means for them to tell an unfolding story to the researcher (and, in fact, themselves). Drawing on these representations, the author describes the extended ways in which her interlocutors think about their bodies; from the mingling of substance, needle and skin, outwards, to spaces and places. She argues that a focus on the assemblage of elements which form the event, rather than distinguishing the body from the drug, has the potential to reframe interventions and understandings of drug use. The constraining nature of wider moral and social framings are also present in Mills' paper (2017). In her research, however, rather than the formation of assemblages associated with an event, the body itself is the meeting point for non-human actants in the form of HIV and antiretroviral therapies (ARVs). Drawing on the concept of posthumanist performativity, HIV and ARVs are presented as travelling complex pathways in, and within, women's bodies as women navigate the challenging healthcare resources of South Africa. But throughout Mills' paper, biomedical technologies are presented as more than a material body-nonhuman assemblage, and instead must be situated in the broader social and politics landscape.

In contrast, Lynch and Cohn (2017) take as their starting point a topic frequently reduced to the broader politics of life – blood donation. They argue that the exclusion of the routine, material aspects of blood donation in much research masks a hidden multiplicity of concepts. Through ethnographic analysis that focuses on the meeting of non-humans and parts of the body, they suggest blood is something that is 'made' only when it leaves the body. Donated blood, they argue, is not simply extracted but constructed through the process of donation, with different material practices making various 'kinds' of blood. Lynch and Cohn argue against altruistic framings of donation to suggest that it is the increasing depersonalisation and reconstitutions of these different bloods that give the resulting substances their biomedical value. Like Mills and Dennis, such work not only foregrounds the encounters and relations between the human and the non-human, but speaks to the wider values, political concerns and conceptual framings of public health approaches.

Using medical technology itself to draw out people's wider values, concerns and framings, the final research paper in this collection comprises a thought experiment to provoke discussion and reflection. Lehoux and colleagues (Lahoux, Williams-Jones, Grimard, & Proulx, 2017) introduce a group of participants to a hypothetical technology aimed at reducing school drop-out rates; a 'smart sweater' able to provide bio-psycho-feedback to the wearer about their mental state and cognitive functioning. Drawing on the increasing popularity of self-monitoring technologies and performance enhancement substances, this case study was used to provoke moral debate about the legitimacy of such an intervention and the tension between autonomy and social coercion. While many of the other papers indirectly point to ethical standpoints and movements arising from posthumanism, this paper explicitly illustrates how posthuman approaches may draw out the moral positioning of interlocutors themselves.

Finally, an engaging commentary by Svendsen (2017) provides a personal reflection on her ethnographic work linking neonatal care with experiments conducted on pigs. Her work not only concerns how these two field sites are connected – the research done on the animals translating to interventions conducted on frail newborns – but the way they become mutually entangled. People, concepts and even substances regularly cross from one site to another such that pigs move from being an outlandish subject on the edge of public health to one of central importance. Pigs, neonates, care and experimentation are drawn together to once again destabilise notions of a public health as being solely concerned with human populations. In her commentary, and throughout the other contributions to this special issue, the concept of 'human being' is substituted for accounts of 'being human'. It is perhaps this that ultimately speaks to, and might reinforce, a critical public health; one that recognises health as an emergent quality of relations, but that those relations are ever changing, diverse and often surprising.

References

Bostrom, N. (2005). Transhumanist values. *Journal of Philosophical Research, 30*, 3–14.

Braidotti, R. (2015). *The Posthuman*. Cambridge: Polity Press.

Carrithers, M., Collins, S., & Lukes, S. (1985). *The category of the person: Anthropology, philosophy, history*. Cambridge: Cambridge University Press.

Dennis, F. (2017). The injecting 'event': Harm reduction beyond the human. *Critical Public Health, 27*, 337–349.

Diamond, N. (2013). *Between skins: The body in psychoanalysis-contemporary developments*. Chichester: Wiley.

Elder-Vass, D. (2015). Disassembling actor-network theory. *Philosophy of the Social Sciences, 45*, 100–121.

Engel, G. L. (1977). The need for a new medical model. *Science, 196*, 129–136.

Friese, C., & Nuyts, N. (2017). Posthumanist critique and human health: How nonhumans (could) figure in public health research. *Critical Public Health, 27*, 303–313.

Garnett, E. (2017). Enacting toxicity: Epidemiology and the study of air pollution for public health. *Critical Public Health, 27*, 325–336.

Habermas, J., & Levin, T. Y. (1982). The entwinement of myth and enlightenment: Re-reading dialectic of enlightenment. *New German Critique, 26*, 13–30.

Haraway, D. (1991). Cyborg manifesto: Science, technology, and socialist-feminism in the late twentieth century. In D. Haraway (Ed.), *Simians, Cyborgs and women: The reinvention of nature* (pp. 149–181). New York, NY: Routledge.

Helmreich, S. (2015). *Sounding the limits of life: Essays in the anthropology of biology and beyond*. Princeton, NJ: Princeton University Press.

Jay, M. (1984). *Marxism and totality: The adventures of a concept from Lukács to Habermas*. Berkeley: University of California Press.

Jensen, C. B., & Winthereik, B. R. (2013). *Monitoring movements in development aid: Recursive partnerships and infrastructures*. Cambridge, Mass: MIT Press.

Kohn, E. (2013). *How forests think: Toward an anthropology beyond the human*. Berkeley: University of California Press.

Koplan, J. P., Bond, T. C., Merson, M. H., Reddy, K. S., Rodriguez, M. H., Sewankambo, N. K., & Wasserheit, J. N. (2009). Towards a common definition of global health. *The Lancet, 373*, 1993–1995.

Krieger, N. (1992). Re: Who made John Snow a hero? *American Journal of Epidemiology, 135*, 450–451. [letter]

Landecker, H. (2016). Antibiotic resistance and the biology of history. *Body & Society, 22*, 19–52.

Latour, B. (2005). *Reassembling the social: An introduction to actor-network-theory*. Oxford: Oxford University Press.

Law, J. (2004). And if the global were small and noncoherent? Method, complexity, and the baroque. *Environment and Planning D: Society and Space, 22*, 13–26.

Lehoux, P., Williams-Jones, B., Grimard, D., & Proulx, S. (2017). Technologies of the self in public health: Insights from public deliberations on cognitive and behavioural enhancement. *Critical Public Health, 27*, 373–383.

Lynch, R., & Cohn, S. (2017). Beyond the person: The construction and transformation of blood as a resource. *Critical Public Health, 27*, 362–372.

McNamee, M. J., & Edwards, S. D. (2006). Transhumanism, medical technology and slippery slopes. *Journal of Medical Ethics, 32*, 513–518.

Mills, E. (2017). Biopolitical precarity in the permeable body: The social lives of people, viruses and their medicines. *Critical Public Health, 27*, 350–361.

Morris, B. (1991). *Western conceptions of the individual*. Oxford: Berg.

Oudshoorn, N. (2003). *Beyond the natural body: An archaeology of sex hormones*. New York, NY: Routledge.

Redfield, P. (2013). *Life in crisis: The ethical journey of doctors without borders*. Berkeley: University of California Press.

Rock, M. (2017). Who or what is "the public" in critical public health? Reflections on posthumanism and anthropological engagements with one health. *Critical Public Health, 27*, 314–324.

Rorty, R. (1984). Habermas and Lyotard on post-modernity. *Praxis International, 4*, 32–44.

Scott-Baumann, A. (2009). *Ricoeur and the hermeneutics of suspicion*. London: Continuum/Bloomsbury Publishing.

Svendsen, M. (2017). Pigs in public health. *Critical Public Health, 27*, 384–390

Tirosh-Samuelson, H. (2012). Transhumanism as a secularist faith. *Zygon®, 47*, 710–734.

Turing, A. M. (1950). Computing machinery and intelligence. *Mind, 59*, 433–460.

Will, C. (2017). On difference and doubt as tools for critical engagement with public health. *Critical Public Health, 27*, 293–302.

Wolfe, C. (2010). *What is Posthumanism?* Minneapolis, MN: University of Minnesota Press.

Simon Cohn
Rebecca Lynch

On difference and doubt as tools for critical engagement with public health

Catherine M. Will

ABSTRACT

This paper argues that critical public health should reengage with public health as practice by drawing on versions of Science and Technology Studies (STS) that 'de-centre the human' and by seeking alternative forms of critique to work inspired by Foucault. Based on close reading of work by Annemarie Mol, John Law, Vicky Singleton and others, I demonstrate that these authors pursue a conversation with Foucault but suggest new approaches to studying contemporary public health work in different settings. Proposing that we 'doubt' both the unity of public health and its effects, I argue that this version of STS opens up a space to recognise multiplicity; to avoid idealising what is being criticised; and to celebrate or care for public health practices as part of critique. Finally I oppose the view that considering technologies, materials and microbes leads to micro-level analysis or political neutrality, and suggest that it allows us to reframe studies of public health to account for inequalities and to draw attention to weak or retreating states, active markets and the entangled relations of humans and non-humans across the world.

Introduction

Current discussion of the concept of posthumanism invokes a wide range of authors, including those who 'de-centre the human' as a result of their interest in technologies and materials. Generally located within Science and Technology Studies (STS), the work of Annemarie Mol, John Law and Vicky Singleton addresses the entangled relations between humans and non-humans of different kinds, including public health technologies and those who use them. In this paper I explore the theoretical and methodological value of such work for those developing critical perspectives on public health. Rather than weapons to use against contemporary public health I argue this literature offers us tools for new engagement. In the paper these tools will be summarised as different forms of doubt: doubt in the unity of public health, doubt in its effects, and doubt in the strength of the state that is its traditional sponsor. Before expanding on these arguments, I will start by locating them in relation to current interest in 'posthumanist' theory and previous work that draws on Michel Foucault.

Like STS, posthumanist theory is reflected in only a scattering of references in *Critical Public Health*. In a recent commentary Rock, Degeling, and Blue (2014) pull together diverse theoretical traditions including 'Actor Network Theory' (associated by the authors with Bruno Latour, Michel Callon and John Law) and the concept of 'enactment' (associated with Mol's book *The Body Multiple*). In her broader account of 'post anthropocentric thought' Braidotti (2013) similarly draws heavily on STS though she makes more reference to feminist work associated with Donna Haraway, anthropologies of technology and Foucauldian studies of biopower under this heading. Though both Foucault and these authors see human subjects as emerging in relation to techniques and practices, one could challenge the inclusion of Foucauldian work as part of STS, which is as interested in the 'making' of objects as subjects (though cautious about working with a strict division between the two). A more serious problem with Braidotti's characterisation of the literature is her criticism of 'STS' as doing only 'analytical post-humanism'. She argues that work she understands as 'STS' fails to offer 'sustained political analysis of the posthuman condition' because of the 'high degree of political neutrality it expresses about the posthuman predicament' (p. 42). This is a crucial point for readers of this journal and others seeking critical perspectives but I do not recognise it as a good description of the work of Mol. Braidotti makes only one brief reference to Mol's work, but I argue Mol and others like her are important representatives of this tradition if we wish to develop new critical work in public health, and that they are rarely neutral.

I start this paper with a close examination of the relationship between Mol and Foucault, who is one of the most commonly cited theorists in this journal (with more than double the number of citations as Bourdieu, Giddens or Marx). A simple reason for this may of course be the emphasis Foucault puts on public health in his writing. Though suspicious of its disciplinary effects Foucault gives great importance to a field that often appears a poor relation to clinical medicine. Charting the close relationship between public health interventions and the growth in liberal government, he helps give coherence to activities as diverse as tackling sanitation or pollution and asking people to change what they eat, drink or do. As the work of Armstrong (1993, 2014) shows, though public health may increasingly focus on 'behaviour change' historical continuities can be identified in the use of concepts or practices of 'risk' 'surveillance' and 'discipline'. Where Foucault showed these informing material interventions such as architecture and urban planning, these may now be explored in relation to other technologies of modern public health including leaflets, websites and apps. Such interventions may then be seen as expressions of both population thinking and what one author calls a 'deeply punitive medico-moral discourse' (McNaughton, 2011) that is often assumed rather than shown to have disciplining effects on the individual.

Though Foucault offers powerful weapons for analysing the practices of public health as part of what he calls 'advanced liberalism', his historical account necessarily makes broad links across different locations and times. The very first argument I take from Mol is that such fields are rarely as monolithic as might appear. This argument is clearly made in *The Body Multiple*, which is probably the most influential of Mol's works to date. Explaining how this book and her *Logic of Care* develops a conversation with Foucault, I argue that doubting the unity of public health – attending (in Mol's terms) to its multiplicity – is likely to produce quite different accounts from work that starts from Foucault's account of governmentality. In my second section, I draw on a broader range of work by Mol and her collaborators to develop doubts about the consequences of public health in practice. We should acknowledge not just that such interventions may be diverse, but that their effects cannot be simply read off from the interventions or policy. Effects have to be identified through studies of practices, which draw together and create subjects, objects, humans and non-humans in ways that go beyond surveillance and discipline. Moving across studies of technologies for providing clean water and heart health in specific communities, I elaborate on the development of this strand of STS as a way of attending to the different and often unequal outcomes of public health interventions. In my final section I suggest that the multiple and relational ontologies of these authors can inform new forms of critical engagement with the local and global inequalities that shape contemporary public health work. Studies of 'healthy' eating for humans and animals, and of commercial products promising clean water or good nutrition, require attention to the relative weakness of different states and the powerful networks that make global markets, as well as the differences they create between citizens and consumers in different locations. Attending to these complexities does not make for neutrality, but allows for *more* critical responses to some public health initiatives and also encourages us to celebrate, even ally, with others that are open to diverse experiences and situations.

Reading Mol's *Body Multiple* and *Logic of Care* as a conversation with Foucault

Mol's *The Body Multiple* (2002) is a major contribution to studies of bodies and their diseases, clinical knowledges and practices. Written in parallel texts, it counterpoises observations of the way in which atherosclerosis is 'enacted' in a hospital with theoretical reflection on the meaning and use of such ethnographic studies. Taking aim at a perhaps comfortable division of labour between a humanist medical sociology that documents 'illness experience' and a medical concern with 'disease', Mol shows how different specialisms produce or 'enact' different bodies and versions of atherosclerosis through practices such as talk with patients, observation, laboratory analysis and surgery. Where medical sociology documents patient voices, Mol puts the practices, tools and techniques of the hospital at the centre of her discussion. In developing a new account of 'clinical work' and the ways it produces disease, she explicitly built on the writing of Foucault, especially his *Birth of the Clinic* (1976).

Mol also offers numerous reflections about points of similarity and difference between her writing and work inspired by Foucault. Citing Armstrong (1988), whose discussion of public health also drew extensively on Foucault, she suggests a common interest in the material practice of medicine and the ways in which this shapes understanding of the body, for example the development of pathology out of the organisation of eighteenth-century hospitals. However, Mol suggests – putting her own work into Foucault's historical framework – that medicine may no longer relate to pathology as foundational. Her own approach is to 'doubt' (Mol, 2002, p. 47) this rather than argue about the ill effects that might follow.

Foucault's historical vision meant he tended to characterise 'regimes' of knowing as replacing each other over long periods. Mol's identification of 'multiplicity' within the hospital suggests different regimes can and do coexist in the present, though they may certainly compete. Indeed she sees 'clinical' ways of working as under threat. Though Mol insists the book 'does not engage in criticism' she does argue:

> Where a so-called scientific rationale (be it that of pathology, pathophysiology or, most likely at the moment, that of clinical epidemiology) is brought into practice, with sufficient effort it may well come to dominate the other modes that are already at work. But this does not so much improve medicine as impoverish it. (p. 182)

Why does Mol wish to defend clinical medicine – a very different project from that of Foucault? The answer is that unlike other ways of doing medicine she suggests clinical work is willing to live with the kinds of multiplicity that she identifies. Clinical ways of working start from patient histories and work through 'adaptable subjective evaluation rather than requiring objectified figures' (p. 183). Mol does not need to go back to patient stories or perspectives to find ways to value individual experience, but sees sensitivity to difference as emerging in the practices of (some) clinical staff.

Though claiming to eschew criticism, Mol is unapologetic about having a political message. She questions versions of medical reform that emphasise 'patient autonomy' and position patients as a consumer or citizen whose 'will and desires are supposed to be set, predetermined and clear' (Mol, 2002, p. 169), seeking to make space for more nuanced experiences and for caring relations. Moving away from a 'politics of who' she calls for 'politics of what' that can attend to dissonant versions of 'the good life' 'the diverging and coexisting enactments of the good' (p. 176). Clinical epidemiology fails to do this, in her account, for 'instead of being staged in a theatre of discords, differences are flattened out onto a spreadsheet,' (p. 174).

In her more recent and less theoretical book – *Logic of Care* – Mol (2008) develops this argument. Though references to Foucault are here relegated to endnotes, her links to him are arguably stronger for she chooses to focus not on the object (disease) but on the formation of subjects by different 'logics' in health care, highlighting practices that enact people as 'citizens', 'consumers' or 'patients'. Again she aligns with a 'clinical' view that approaches people as patients needing care, rather than citizens or consumers who exercise choice. This book thus draws a distinction between the 'patient' and 'citizen', where Foucault's discussion of medicine in the advanced liberal state tends to collapse the two.

Where does this leave critical public health? I have noted Mol's concern about the rise of 'clinical epidemiology' – but it seems to make little sense to ask public health practices to become more sensitive to 'patients' as individuals. Public health work promises to preserve and improve health for a collective, and draws fundamentally on epidemiology as the science of populations. We cannot just ask it to be more like clinical medicine. But we should be prepared to recognise that it is 'multiple' in practice. To apply Mol's thinking from *Body Multiple* or *Logic of Care* would then involve looking for different ways of doing public health, and doubting whether any single one dominates. Indeed this approach is evident in two areas of research where Mol has worked with other authors, including writing with Law on foot and mouth disease (based on work by Law and Singleton),[1] and secondly in collaborative research on eating practices. I return to these examples later, but will first draw on an earlier piece by Mol written with Marianne De Laet, which has a slightly different approach, and work by Vicky Singleton, to propose a second type of 'doubt' as a tool for a post-Foucauldian critical public health.

Doubting and loving

In this section I consider how Mol has addressed public health explicitly, in a classic paper co-authored with Marianne De Laet. The paper has an unusual form for it is presented as a celebration of a Zimbabwean water pump as public health intervention (De Laet & Mol, 2000). Like clinical work the 'bush pump' is tolerant of difference, and thrives on it. Its parsimonious design means it is meant to be easy to install and repair in different rural sites across Zimbabwe. It is cheap, attractive and welcoming, embodying a quiet reproach to public health technologies that are too rigid to allow local adaptation. It is also 'public' in at least two senses, being produced without patent and promoted as part of government sanitation policy: De Laet and Mol argue that its spread helps draw together the Zimbabwean nation. The authors ask us to accept the pump as an actor, but their primary interest is not identifying pump's disciplinary effects, nor critique.

> In the critical tradition scholars approve or disapprove of technologies, people, situations, arguments. This makes sense if there are clear-cut points of contrast from which to judge. But this isn't always the case. (p. 253)

Rather than offer contrasts, they choose instead to describe a single technology, to 'be moved by' the pump, to 'love' it.

The paper demonstrates the STS preference for putting technologies at the centre of analysis, but it becomes a story about the pump as an effect of work by communities that adopt it. The authors insist that for the technology to spread and be useful it has to be flexible (they talk about its 'fluidity'). Pumps must insert themselves itself into a wider set of relationships that mediate their effects. They note for example that the pump's status as a public health technology rests on demonstrations of reduced counts of *E. coli* bacteria in water produced by the pump. Yet these reductions are always relative (a bush pump may be better than the alternative even when the *E. coli* load remains high) and the relation between *E. coli* and health also 'depends not only on the number of *E. coli* but also on who(se) they are' (De Laet & Mol, 2000, p. 243). Local people may harmonise with the micro-organisms in a well that would cause illness in a stranger.

So far the paper appears to fit with a posthuman framing that pays attention to relations between materials, animals and people and celebrates a fluid object. 'Our actor, the Bush Pump, goes to show once again that actors do not have to be humans' (2000, p. 253). Yet the pump is not the only hero. For, their story about the distributed achievement of the water pump is learned in part from a man characterised as its 'modest innovator'. In celebrating the bush pump the paper also celebrates the man who designed it and continues to negotiate for its use – a man called Peter Morgan. Morgan is presented as a careful student of the communities within which the bush pump might find a home. Though hoping in public health parlance to achieve 'behaviour change' he narrates his work as making the technology ready to fit in with existing practices and relations in these communities. The pump is designed to be appreciated. Where a Foucauldian account might well narrate this as a technology that brings the state into everyday life, Morgan is clear that such top-down interventions can fail, and must work hard to generate attachments that ensure their use.

> In Zimbabwe, village level participation is actively encouraged in all water and sanitation schemes. It is now well established that without this participation, communities cannot generate the commitment for maintenance as they do when they are involved. (Morgan quoted De Laet & Mol, 2000, p. 234)

The final part of the paper acknowledges the times when a 'community' fails to materialise around a pump, or the pump proves 'too weak … [or] insufficiently attractive to become a centre' (p. 245). Some pumps are not maintained and fall into disrepair. Others enter private ownership, being maintained by a small number of families. 'Such a change might make rural Zimbabwe look different, made up of units that are different from those the governments has been seeking to reinforce,' (p. 246). Even so, Morgan continues to embrace the strategy of abandoning control, allowing for surprises, involving and making room for users. His visits to water pumps are not for maintenance, but to learn from the way the pumps have evolved in the wild.

The attempt to preserve openness about the likely effects of a technological intervention is characteristic of STS, and is the second kind of 'doubt' I want to recommend for critical public health. For all its celebration of the bush pump, De Laet and Mol make space for the possibility that the pump will have very few or unexpected local effects. As others have noted, this is actually a relatively common outcome for public health interventions (Cohn, 2014; Lindsay, 2010). Redfield (2016) notes that access to clean water in Zimbabwe is still a problem. As discussed later, he describes the development of new commercial technologies as a result, which are framed much more around individuals or families than the communities that were so important in the bush pump story. We should not assume that even such a loveable technology will be embraced in practice.

A second example helps illustrate the need for doubt about the outcomes of public health, but makes some important additional points about how this should inform critical work. Though not a direct collaborator of Mol, Vicky Singleton has frequently written together with John Law, and her work develops many of the same ideas as his work and Mol's. In a particularly useful piece for this paper, she explicitly addresses the difference between an account of community public health that starts from Foucault and one grounded in this strand of STS. Sharing Mol's interest in practices, but refusing to celebrate them on this occasion, Singleton (2005) starts with a policy document *Saving Lives* that called for public health to involve communities, to tackle inequalities and 'empower' lay people in England and Wales. As she observes, an avowedly Foucauldian analysis of this document starts by drawing attention to the new forms of discipline and surveillance that this may involve.

> Attempts to 'emancipate' or 'empower' marginalised groups … based on humanistic, neo-liberal principles, may be regarded as ever more complex ways of defining, regulating and normalising the members of such groups. (Petersen & Lupton, 1996, quoted in Singleton, 2005, p. 780)

However expressing her own readiness to appreciate public health interventions Singleton argues:

> The New Public Health Policy can be seen as a move in the right direction for health care. It is an attempt to develop health policy and practices sensitive to the complexity of the relationships between the state and individuals and to the multiple meanings and causes of 'good health'. (Singleton, 2005, p. 774)

Her reading of the policy document is thus full of promise but this does not mean she is not prepared to be critical. In an ethnographic study of a community cardio-pulmonary resuscitation project in a rural area of England, she observes that people may certainly be excluded and stigmatised for their failure to participate. Sounding like a Foucauldian, she observes 'active citizens are being made good and inactive citizens are constructed as "stupid and ignorant", selfish and bad' (p. 778). But she argues that these effects are made in the practices or enactment of the policy rather than necessarily contained within it. It is the transposition of the policy into the material networks of community action, defibrillators, village halls, tea, biscuits, cars and volunteers that creates such exclusions. Practices appear as less creative, more conventional and more conservative than the policy itself. This is a provocative claim, and opens up intriguing possibilities for the study of public health as not only internally divided, but also defensive and often unsuccessful. In making this proposal, I feel close to Bell and Green's (2016) call for more 'nuance and specificity' in accounts of public health as responsibilisation within a broader set of processes of neoliberalisation. In my final section I will pick up this concern using some observations by Mol herself on the limits of the 'neoliberal critique', as one which overlaps but is certainly not identical with a Foucauldian one, using discussions of 'good food' for animals and humans to illustrate the argument.

Weak states and private/public health

Foucault's critique of public health is tied up with its close connection with the state, which frames a population and helps develop the practices of advanced liberalism. As Bell and Green (2016) observe, the term 'neoliberal' may be used to describe governmental processes where the focus is on the creation of specific subjects, but also invokes privatisation, the expansion of global markets and the rolling back of the state. I have already discussed how Mol may draw different conclusions from those analyses of public health that see it as a form of governmentality. In this final section I want to explore how we can account for the expansion of commercial activity in the context of weak or retreating states and local and global inequalities.

Mol's most recent work on eating proceeds by a combination of identifying differences (as in *The Body Multiple*) and celebrating particularity (as in the bush pump). Together with several collaborators she has pursued ethnographic studies of eating practices and interventions in settings including nursing homes and the offices of dieticians and health coaches. They contrast different ways of 'doing' nutritional advice that simultaneously avoid a different critical confrontation – and its dismissal of situated knowledges – and appreciate the absence of such critique in informants' practices. Writing with Else Vogel, for example, Mol observes that some professionals encourage people to cultivate pleasure in eating, 'crafting situations and meals that give joy' rather than seeking ever-stronger self-discipline (Vogel & Mol, 2014). They hope to support such efforts which are perhaps the public health equivalent of clinical sensitivity, to 'strengthen and sharpen the theoretical creativity of our informants and help their insights to travel beyond their daily practices' (p. 306).

Vogel and Mol (2014) explicitly address the question of whether they have been 'critical' enough in ways that attend to local practices and the networks in which they are embedded. First they note the weakness of public health – its enforced modesty if you like. Public health workers confront food practices that are shaped by intensive marketing of unhealthy and processed food, where governments seem unable or unwilling to act. All that remains for dieticians is 'the possibility of addressing consumers and urging them to make healthy food choices' (p. 306). But the injunction to listen to your body, to embrace rather than resist the pleasures of eating, may support those markets.

> None of this is beyond criticism. Enjoy your food resonates with the advertisement messages of food industries, which makes it easy to be misused. What is more, not all possible food pleasures are being endorsed. Calm enjoyment is being fostered and wild ecstasy is not. (p. 314)

Nodding to the disciplinary critique of public health they acknowledge 'a very thin line between liberating the pleasures of the body and imposing yet more obligations on the caring self', (p. 315), but they say they want to support what seems to them a better version of public health than some others. 'It is just too easy to write in a social science journal that encouraging people to take pleasure from their food is nothing but another neoliberal disciplining strategy' (p. 315).

This example is helpful to show how critical engagement with public health may involve new positions that are not simply set against 'government', 'commerce' or an alliance of the two described as 'neoliberal'. This argument is also made by Redfield (2016) in his discussion of new ways of providing clean water in Zimbabwe, developed as part of his own critical appreciation of the bush pump article. Redfield gives us the example of the LifeStraw®, the product of a Norwegian firm based in Switzerland, which he sees as a partial response to the weakness of the nation state. The LifeStraw® he tells us is a product of commercial efforts to find new organisational forms that 'mix ethics with finance'. Though it is initially sold it may also be given away, while the company makes money from trading the 'carbon' saved if families no longer boil water to kill bacteria – in a global carbon reduction market. Like Vogel and Mol, Redfield wants to resist any easy criticism of this scheme as 'neoliberal' (Redfield, 2016, p. 16). He sees in the company an orientation to people as consumers, which makes them attentive to their needs. 'To be successful humanitarian goods must recognise their users, adjusting to the reality of their worlds even as they seek to change them' (p. 15). Like Mol's sense of the clinical, Redfield finds sensitivity to difference in commercial design. He wonders if it is possible to see in the case a positive alternative vision of water infrastructures that keeps in view the specificities of the product, the limited action of the state in which it is distributed, and the promise as well as pitfalls of the market.

Redfield treads the tight rope of appreciating a commercial product without appearing its dupe, but this allows him to extend his analysis beyond the local practical accomplishment of a set of relations, to include more global networks. Two final examples show how Mol and her colleagues might do something similar, moving away from 'micro-level' analysis of relations to connections across national borders. The first presents itself as a debate with Jane Bennett, a key author in studies of 'new material-ism'. Picking up on Bennett's interest in fatty acids known as omega-3 as an example of the interrelations between objects and humans (see Bennett, 2010), Abrahamsson, Nertoni, Ibanez-Martin and Mol seek to address a number of issues. They acknowledge her identification of omega-3 as an object that alters human mood and cognition, but question her way of attending to 'science' in order to substantiate her claim (Abrahamsson, Bertoni, Mol, & Martin, 2015). For example, instead of focusing on supposedly gen-eralised results, they argue it is important to pay attention to 'materials and methods' sections and the research practices they unfold. In fact, the studies Bennett relies on to make the argument that omega-3 is important were conducted in prisons because of the easy dietary control they afford; while the studies can show correlations in changes in nutrition and behaviour for an already deprived and malnourished group, they are not so easily extrapolated to 'humans' in general. The authors go on to decry the lack of attention to wider issues behind omega-3 use in rich countries. The production of omega-3 is reliant on a scarce natural resource, they observe, and its conversion into nutritional supplements involves the export of fish from the global South. As well as smoothing over the contribution of nutritional inequal-ities to the production of evidence, 'Bennett talks about omega-3 without directly concerning herself with such contentious issues as the inequalities between well-fed and under-nourished people or the startling depletions of fish stocks worldwide' (Abrahamsson et al., 2015, p. 13). While sharing Bennett's interest in material–human relations, they use the focus on 'relationality' and difference to put politics explicitly into the discussion of nutritional supplements.

The final material for this theoretical debate is pigswill, an unpromising topic perhaps but an impor-tant part of the story of the foot and mouth outbreak studied by Vicky Singleton and John Law. Pigswill is scarcely commercial and never branded. It is not produced through flows of materials from the South to the North like omega-3, but from the 'metabolic surplus' existing in rich countries with significant volumes of food waste that can be recycled as animal feed. In seeking to describe its politics Law and Mol (2008) narrate pigswill in posthuman terms, for it mixes humans, animals, microbes and machines. One story might then be about pigswill as a risk to public health. Though countries try to control the movements of meat and microbes across their borders, they do not always succeed. If infected meat finds its way into the food chain, careless use of pigswill made from food waste may allow the infection to spread to live animals. The failure to boil pigswill on just one farm can be blamed for an outbreak of the disease and the decision to slaughter millions of animals. Yet, Law and Mol demonstrate how attention to a mundane object can open up more critical perspectives on state and market failures, global inequalities and trade flows. 'Boiling pigswill was a political technique that, in a region of plenty, respected and helped to limit food scarcity on a world wide scale' (Law & Mol, 2008, p. 141). Though useful in the context of weak borders, pigswill used local materials otherwise defined as 'waste'. It thus had some advantages over feeding pigs on meal derived from crops produced through 'industrial agriculture', with effects including pollution and reworking of the landscape. In this paper the authors therefore use a relational approach to debate the different 'goods' of public health as well as the com-plexities of human/non human relations.

Tools not weapons

In this synthesis, I have drawn on relatively scattered work to propose new tools for critical engagement with public health. I have argued that Mol, Law, Singleton and others in STS offer ways of doing social science that encourage us to grapple with difference and resist some of the pleasures of denuncia-tion. Criticising some characterisations of this literature, I suggest that these authors should be read as attempting a conversation with Foucault and his followers. Rather than offer a straight alternative, they respond to and develop his analysis, and relate carefully to the very idea of 'critical work'. Like other authors in STS – including Haraway (1991) and Latour (2004) – they hope 'no longer to debunk but to protect and care' (Latour, 2004, p. 232). But where Latour (2004) calls for authors in STS to 'review their equipment and training' like every good general', Law (2008) explicitly resists military metaphor. Rather than rearming, in his work and collaborations with Mol and Singleton, Law seeks methods or tools for a different kind of engagement. In this final section I will draw on this broader discussion in STS and previous work in this journal, to summarise the potential of this particular type of posthumanism to inform new accounts of public health.

In this paper I have proposed the work of Mol as a rich source of inspiration for writing on public health. Though we may not always find equivalents for the practices that she celebrates in clinical medicine, we can, like Mol, start from an assumption that public health work is characterised by multiplicity, that it brings together different practices and knowledges. This helps avoid any overly monolithic views of public health or indeed the state or governmental regime – views that would imagine the state as a stable and given entity rather than a dynamic set of contingent practices. In STS relations between knowledge practices, interventions, humans and non-humans are conceived as fragile: it is common to start the analysis with doubts as to whether these networks can be held together across space and time, and whether any practice will have a durable or fixed character (Law, 2008). For example though epidemiology may appear important in accounts of the history of public health it may be useful to characterise different ways of doing epidemiology, or challenges from psychology, marketing or economics. Instead of positioning ourselves as external critical voices, attending to varied practices in the field may allow social scientists to become allies in reimagining public health work. Very similar suggestions have been made by other authors in STS (see Barad, 2007; Haraway, 1991 on the method of diffraction, or Latour, 2007 and Marres & Lezaun, 2011 on material politics), but Mol and Law offer excellent examples of this analytic approach. Not all public health interventions look as 'modest' or as loveable as the bush pump, but Mol may inspire us to go looking for those that are.

The second set of doubts discussed in this paper related to the effects of public health interventions. I suggested that work in STS encourages greater openness about the possible results of public health than expressed by Foucauldian scholars, who can appear quick to assume 'governmental' effects from very diverse interventions (e.g. McNaughton, 2011; Petersen & Lupton, 1996). When they acknowledge uncertainty about whether public health can foster discipline, they may celebrate 'resistance' (e.g. McLean, 2011; McPhail, 2013; Petersen, 1998). In the STS literature unexpected responses to policies or technologies may also be celebrated, for example as forms of creative appropriation or domestication (e.g. Carter, Green, & Thorogood, 2013; Lie & Sørensen, 1996; Silverstone, Hirsch, & Morley, 1992; Kline & Pinch, 1996; Weiner & Will, 2015). Paying attention to resistance, appropriation and domestication may produce more satisfying accounts of the politics of objects than the focus on discipline, but such themes can still reduce the force of that initial doubt about the effects of interventions and the possibility of indifference (Lindsay, 2010). Though not sharing the prominence of De Laet and Mol's bush pump paper, Singleton's commitment to questioning the effects of policy – and readiness to see policy as potentially more sensitive or emancipatory than practice – reminds us to focus on the different ways in which people experience interventions or resist them. While most attention has been on public health 'technologies of the self' as normalising and universalising, some recent work has argued that some groups are found incapable of such self-discipline and subject to more punitive responses, stigma and abjection (e.g. Barcelos, 2014; Thompson & Kumar, 2011). Work on public health can connect powerfully with other scholarship addressing inequalities and injustice (e.g. Tyler, 2013), showing how local negotiations may create exclusions in practice, even when such work starts from analytical openness about the distribution of goods and bads.

In expressing our own willingness to 'love' elements of public health as well as the potential importance of abjection, we might also more readily engage with a range of emotional responses to governmental interventions and the objects that public health makes problematic (including cigarettes and drugs as well as 'unhealthy' foods). Mol's work on healthy eating is a useful reminder that we need to account not only for discipline but also for pleasure, the preferred terrain of the market, but objects also produce emotions like disgust. Though there was not space to develop this argument in detail here, it is worth noting that while STS is cautious about drawing clear lines between subjects and objects, its attention to objects is different from Foucauldian work. As Mol says in defending herself against humanist critics:

> It may well be that … [Actor Network Theory] fails to protect humans from being treated as 'mere things', but it offers something else instead. It opens up the possibility of seeing, hearing, sensing and then analysing the social life of things – and thus of caring about, rather than neglecting them. (Mol, 2010, p. 255)

So far I have elaborated the need for doubt about the results of public health interventions and more attention to their different objects as well as their subjects. In the third section I highlighted an additional effect of focusing on the 'social life of things' that gets too little attention from those who represent STS as politically neutral. While authors like Mol may be careful about offering 'critique' and resist political slogans, politics is unavoidable if we focus attention on technologies and materials for they are hardly ever equally accessible to everyone. In the discussion of eating for pleasure, the LifeStraw, omega-3 and pigswill I have shown that STS engages with diverse public health practices *and* helps explore the global relations that shape human and animal health. In the markets that supply our food and the regulation and movements of microbes and nutrients we find numerous reminders that public health work is subject to pressures beyond the jurisdiction of any single government. Its practices continually negotiate, produce and reproduce inequalities between different subjects and objects, not least in contexts where states appear reluctant or incapable of acting on their populations. This sensibility may be less celebrated in STS than our attention to local practice, but is vital for our understanding of contemporary public health.

Note

1. Though John Law is often associated mainly with Actor Network Theory as a distinct approach, in the last decade he has frequently written with Annemarie Mol and their work has evolved together. He is also a long-term collaborator with a British feminist STS scholar, Vicky Singleton. In several articles these authors explore how foot and mouth disease was identified and managed by the various agencies, experts and stakeholders including farmers living through the foot and mouth outbreak in the UK in 2001. For another example see Singleton's (2010) discussion of farming practices as offering the potential for more sensitive responses to the disease.

Acknowledgements

I am grateful to Rebecca Lynch and Simon Cohn for the encouragement to write this paper, to Simon Carter and Judith Green for the initial invitation to present on the topic at the event celebrating 25 years of the journal, and to participants at that event, my colleague Alison Phipps, and two anonymous reviewers for very helpful comments on previous versions.

Disclosure statement

No potential conflict of interest was reported by the author.

References

Abrahamsson, S., Bertoni, F., Mol, A., & Martin, R. (2015). Living with omega-3: New materialism and enduring concerns. *Environment and Planning D: Society and Space, 33*, 4–19.

Armstrong, D. (1988). Space and time in British general practice. In M. Lock & D. Gorgon (Eds.), *Biomedicine examined* (pp. 659–666). Dordrecht: Kluwer.

Armstrong, D. (1993). Public health spaces and the fabrication of identity. *Sociology, 27*, 393–410.

Armstrong, D. (2014). Actors, patients and agency: A recent history. *Sociology of Health & Illness, 36*, 163–174.

Barad, K. (2007). *Meeting the universe halfway*. Durham, NC: Duke University Press.

Barcelos, C. A. (2014). Producing (potentially) pregnant teen bodies: Biopower and adolescent pregnancy in the USA. *Critical Public Health, 24*, 476–488.

Bell, K., & Green, J. (2016). On the perils of invoking neoliberalism in public health critique. *Critical Public Health, 26*, 239–243.

Bennett, J. (2010). *Vibrant matter: A political ecology of things*. Durham, NC: Duke University Press.

Braidotti, R. (2013). *The posthuman*. Cambridge: Polity Press.

Carter, S., Green, J., & Thorogood, N. (2013). The domestication of an everyday health technology: A case study of electric toothbrushes. *Social Theory & Health, 11*, 344–367.

Cohn, S. (2014). From health behaviours to health practices: An introduction. *Sociology of Health & Illness, 36*, 157–162.

De Laet, M., & Mol, A. (2000). The Zimbabwe bush pump: Mechanics of a fluid technology. *Social Studies of Science, 30*, 225–263.

Foucault, M. (1976). *The birth of the clinic*. London: Tavistock Publications Ltd.

Haraway, D. J. (1991). *Simians, cyborgs, and women: The reinvention of nature*. London: Routledge.

Kline, R., & Pinch, T. (1996). Users as agents of technological change: The social construction of the automobile in the rural United States. *Technology and Culture, 37*, 763–795.

Latour, B. (2004). Why has critique run out of steam? From matters of fact to matters of concern. *Critical Inquiry, 30*, 225–248.

Latour, B. (2007). Turning around politics: A note on Gerard de Vries' paper. *Social Studies of Science, 37*, 811–820.

Law, J. (2008). On sociology and STS. *The Sociological Review, 56*, 623–649.

Law, J., & Mol, A. (2008). Globalisation in practice: On the politics of boiling pigswill. *Geoforum, 39*, 133–143.

Lie, M., & Sørensen, K. H. (1996). *Making technology our own? Domesticating technology into everyday life*. Oslo: Scandinavian University Press.

Lindsay, J. (2010). Healthy living guidelines and the disconnect with everyday life. *Critical Public Health, 20*, 475–487.

Marres, N., & Lezaun, J. (2011). Materials and devices of the public: An introduction. *Economy and Society, 40*, 489–509.

McLean, K. (2011). The biopolitics of needle exchange in the United States. *Critical Public Health, 21*, 71–79.

McNaughton, D. (2011). From the womb to the tomb: Obesity and maternal responsibility. *Critical Public Health, 21*, 179–190.

McPhail, D. (2013). Resisting biopedagogies of obesity in a problem population: Understandings of healthy eating and healthy weight in a Newfoundland and Labrador community. *Critical Public Health, 23*, 289–303.

Mol, A. (2002). *The body multiple*. Durham, NC: Duke University Press.

Mol, A. (2008). *The logic of care: Health and the problem of patient choice*. London: Routledge.

Mol, A. (2010). Actor-network theory: Sensitive terms and enduring tensions. *Kölner Zeitschrift für Soziologie und Sozialpsychologie, 50*, 253–269.

Petersen, A. (1998). The new genetics and the politics of public health. *Critical Public Health, 8*, 59–71.

Petersen, A., & Lupton, D. (1996). *The new public health: Health and self in the age of risk*. London: Sage.

Redfield, P. (2016). Fluid technologies: The Bush Pump, the LifeStraw® and the microworlds of humanitarian design. *Social Studies of Science, 46*, 159–183.

Rock, M., Degeling, C., & Blue, G. (2014). Toward stronger theory in critical public health: Insights from debates surrounding posthumanism. *Critical Public Health, 24*, 337–348.

Silverstone, R., Hirsch, E., & Morley, D. (1992). Information and communication technologies and the moral economy of the household. In R. Silverstone & E. Hirsch (Eds.), *Consuming technologies* (pp. 9–17). London: Routledge.

Singleton, V. (2005). The promise of public health: Vulnerable policy and lazy citizens. *Society and Space, 23*, 771–786.

Singleton, V. (2010). Good farming: Control or care. In A. Mol, I. Moser, & J. Pols (Eds.), *Care in practice: On tinkering in clinics, homes and farms* (pp. 235–256). Bielefeld: Transcript.

Thompson, L., & Kumar, A. (2011). Responses to health promotion campaigns: Resistance, denial and othering. *Critical Public Health, 21*, 105–117.

Tyler, I. (2013). *Revolting subjects: Social abjection and resistance in neoliberal Britain*. London: Zed Books.

Vogel, E., & Mol, A. (2014). Enjoy your food: On losing weight and taking pleasure. *Sociology of Health & Illness, 36*, 305–317.

Weiner, K., & Will, C. (2015). Materiality matters: Blurred boundaries and the domestication of functional foods. *BioSocieties, 10*, 194–212.

Posthumanist critique and human health: how nonhumans (could) figure in public health research

Carrie Friese and Nathalie Nuyts

ABSTRACT

This paper uses bibliometric analysis and critical discourse analysis to explore the rise in research involving nonhumans in public health, and the potential contribution of posthumanist social theory to this growing body of public health scholarship. There has been a sudden and rather marked increase in research and writing on animals, zoonoses and/or the 'One-health' paradigm within public health journals since 2006. Indeed 'One-health' rather than 'posthumanism' holds together research involving nonhumans of various kinds – from viruses to animals – within the discipline. Advocates of the 'One-health' paradigm argue that human and animal health must be integrated through joining the research, training and care practices of human and animal medicine. By mapping the terrain of public health research involving non-human species, we consider how and where posthumanist theory could be productively drawn upon to contribute to both critical and applied research involving nonhumans within public health. We specifically ask how the posthumanist insight to 'follow the nonhumans' would raise new questions and analytics for this research area.

Introduction

There is a growing literature in the social sciences and humanities that explores the salience of nonhumans of various kinds for social life, as this special issue on posthumanism attests to. Posthumanism is a broad and even conflicting area of social theory that seeks to understand how humans are made in tandem with nonhumans of varying kinds, such that separating out humans from the world is problematized. However, public health research has not engaged with the posthumanist scholarship to date. We conducted a search of the terms 'posthuman' and 'public health' in Web of Science, and found only two entries; both articles were published in *Critical Public Health* and were written by the same lead author (Rock, 2013; Rock, Degeling, & Blue, 2014). As a point of comparison, a search in Web of Science for 'posthuman' within the social sciences and humanities resulted in 587 articles published between 2010 and 2014. That said public health *is* researching the ways in which non-human animals and other kinds of non-human agents (such as microbes or viruses) are embroiled in human health. So there is at least some overlap between posthumanism in the social sciences and humanities, and public health research concerned with nonhumans. To consider these spaces of shared interest and the potential for productive dialogue, this article starts with reviewing the literature at the intersection of non-human species and public health using bibliometric analysis and critical discourse analysis. We ask where and how nonhumans figure within public health research today and historically. The aim of this review is to provide an overview to the themes or topics addressed within the public health literature focused on nonhumans. Based on this analysis we consider how posthumanist theory could productively contribute to these areas of public health research into the future.

This paper builds directly upon Rock et al.'s (2014) argument that posthumanist theory is relevant for public health. Towards that end, Rock, Degeling and Blue have provided a synthetic review of the posthumanist literature, tracing it through post-structuralism generally and science and technology studies (STS) in particular. Their goal is to introduce public health to this theory, as they argue it is relevant to research regarding zoonotic infectious diseases, toxins and other environmental contaminants as well as the healthy and unhealthy consequences of pet populations.

The goal of this paper is the inverse. We map how nonhumans currently figure within public health research. Through this mapping we ask if, where and how posthumanist theory could productively contribute to existing research agendas within public health. We start with a brief review of the posthumanist literature as it relates to this article. We then discuss our use of bibliometric analysis in combination with critical discourse analysis, and present our findings based upon this analysis. We demonstrate that the 'One-health' paradigm is providing the theoretical basis for research involving nonhumans in public health research today. One-health is a term that is used to reorganize the relationships between human medicine and animal veterinary medicine, so that these two medical fields speak more to one another in both knowledge and practice. We conclude by considering why public health is turning to One-health, and what posthumanist theory could contribute in this context. We argue that the posthumanist injunction to 'follow the nonhumans around' would raise new questions and analytics for this research area. In particular, this could be productively entwined with existing practices in both critical public health that explores power relationships and social epidemiology that explores relationalities between humans and things, such that posthumanism could extend not only critique in public health, but also more applied practices.

Background to posthumanism

Rock et al. (2014) have provided an excellent discussion of the posthumanist literature for a public health audience. They note that humanism posited an intrinsic value for human life, and a universal capacity amongst people to be moral and rational. Humanism is therefore an important achievement in many respects. But Rock, Degeling and Blue contend that our imbrication with technologies, in particular, has required critiquing some aspects of humanism today, which they do through post-structuralism specifically. Rock, Degeling and Blue contend that Pierre Bourdieu was a post-structuralist who revitalized humanism, while Michel Foucault was a post-structuralist who showed how the notion of the human is itself historically contingent. Rock, Degeling and Blue then trace how post-structuralism has been taken up in some uniquely posthumanist ways since. This includes non-representational theories in geography, which allow us to understand meaning-making in ways that take a more-than-human and more-than-textual world seriously. This also includes actor network theory in STS, which has (in)famously argued that nonhumans must also be understood as agentic. Rock, Degeling and Blue then provide an introduction to other concepts from these fields which may be useful to public health researchers. This includes the idea that purportedly natural things like diseases need to be socially and materially 'enacted' (Mol, 2002) and that agency is relationally distributed across humans and nonhumans through 'meshwork' (Ingold, 2011). Rock, Degeling and Blue conclude that there is space for productive dialogue between public health and anthrozoology, which focuses on the interactions between humans and nonhumans through primatology and ethological perspectives.

Building upon the review of posthumanism offered by Rock, Degeling and Blue, the background section of this article has more modest goals. It is meant to provide necessary context for understanding how and why we selected the search terms that we did in conducting our bibliometric analysis, and what is left out as a consequence of these choices. This background also allows us to discuss the specifics of how posthumanism could contribute to existing public health research agendas in the Conclusion, which is based on our analysis of how nonhumans are currently situated in public health research.

The term 'posthumanism' carries some rather different and even conflicting meanings, informed by various strands of thought including post-structuralism, humanism and cybernetics (Wolfe, 2010). On the one hand, posthumanist thought argues that we need to look at the ways in which humans are embroiled, and thereby develop, or 'become' (Haraway, 2008), with other species as well as other non-human things. For example, physical anthropologists are contributing to posthumanist thought by showing that domestication is not something that we humans simply do to other species; humans also show all the physical traits used to demarcate domesticated species, and so we humans have also changed through our interactions with other animal species over time (Cassidy & Mullin, 2007; Leach, 2003). As such, posthumanist critique is, to some extent, part of the 'materialist turn' in the social sciences and humanities, in that it seeks to recoup the animality of humans as embodied and embedded (Wolfe, 2010, p. xv). This strand of posthumanist thought argues that humanism is a discourse that needs to be troubled, despite the important ways in which it has facilitated rights for various oppressed groups of people (Wolfe, 2010). Specifically, it is argued that humanism is based upon an inadequate division between humans and nonhumans (Cubukcu, in press), one that we need to problematize in order to appreciate human interactions with animals, plants and all the other things that we live with on this planet (Wolfe, 2010). It is a divide that we also need to challenge because, in being based on a hierarchy, humanism risks perpetuating rather than ameliorating differences between humans that can in turn perpetuate rather than ameliorate oppression (Cubukcu, in press). Posthumanism has thus sought to intervene in the anthropocentrism of the social sciences and humanities by emphasizing how we as humans socialize with a variety of nonhumans, including other animal species, plants and inanimate objects. We believe that this strand of posthumanist thought has the most relevance to public health.

But there is a different use of the term posthuman, seen particularly within bioethics but also sociology. Here 'posthumanism' or 'transhumanism' is used as part of an argument that humans can and should develop and use biotechnologies in order to improve human bodies (Fuller, 2011; Savulescu & Bostrom, 2009). There is a glorification of science, choice and consumption here that has been consistently silent on issues of power, refusing to consider how fantasies of biological control risk reproducing hierarchies, including gender, sexuality, race, ethnicity, class, nation, citizenship, age and (dis)ability. This version of posthumanism has therefore been critiqued as an extension of humanism (Wolfe, 2010). Largely developing in bioethics, these posthumanists tend to take, as their counter-argument, those who see biotechnologies as eroding an a priori, unified and fundamental human essence, such as Jurgen Habermas (2003) or Francis Fukuyama (2002). We do not believe that this more speculative and futurist area of thought is particularly relevant to public health at present, or to the goals of critique.

Given that there were only two references to 'posthuman' and 'public health' while also knowing that public health research is considering the implications of human–non-human species relations for health, we decided to search for specific topics in public health research where a posthumanist insight could be relevant. This included zoonotic diseases, animals generally and the 'One-health' paradigm. We asked how research in public health is organized, which is topically compatible with posthumanism but that does not reference to this term. We were also interested in considering the relationship, if any, between these areas of research. The animality of humans is therefore our focus in this paper, and we do not engage in the more cybernetic aspects of posthumanism.

Methods

This paper combines bibliometric methods with critical discourse analysis. To start, bibliometric methods have been adopted in this paper to review the public health literature that addresses non-human species in order to provide insights into what main topics are addressed, and how those topics are addressed. The particular method used in this paper – bibliographic coupling in combination with clustering – has been found to be a valid tool for identifying research themes within a large field (Jarneving, 2007).

The bibliometric data for this paper were gathered from the Web of Science Core Collection database. Within the titles, abstracts and keywords of the publications indexed in this database, a search was executed to select out all articles between 1995 and 2014 that used the terms 'zoonosis' OR 'zoonotic'

OR 'animal' OR 'one health' AND 'public health'. The search criterion 'one health' selected articles that fit within the 'One-health' paradigm as well as publications discussing, for example, 'one health care practice'. Therefore, all the publications selected through this criterion were manually cleaned, keeping only those publications that dealt with the 'One-health' paradigm specifically. In total, the search resulted in 7294 publications, which were analysed by means of bibliographic coupling and cluster analysis.

Bibliographic coupling was used to build a visual map based on the overlap in the references cited by the publications. In other words, distance on this map represents the amount of overlap between the references in the bibliographies of the publications. The more similar the topics of texts are, the closer the articles are located in relationship to one another on the map. The analysis was executed in VoS-viewer, a programme developed for the construction and visualization of bibliometric networks, which uses a mapping technique closely related to multidimensional scaling (van Eck, Waltman, Dekker, & van den Berg, 2010). After the bibliographic coupling, the publications were further assigned to exactly one cluster, or a set of closely related nodes (Waltman, van Eck, & Noyons, 2010). Within clusters, co-citation analysis of the bibliographic references shows the most frequently shared texts. These documents are the foundational references for the topical area. Foundational texts were analysed using critical discourse analysis (Jager & Maier, 2009; Wodak & Meyer, 2009).

Based on the bibliographic analysis, we then conducted a closer analysis of the most frequently cited texts in one key cluster using critical discourse analysis (Jager & Maier, 2009; Wodak & Meyer, 2009). The One-health cluster bridges the different substantive areas of focus in the map, and so we wanted to better understand how nonhumans were discussed in these texts. The question we asked when reading these texts was: how are non-human species represented generally and in relationship to public health specifically in this document? In addition, we also conducted a close reading and critical discourse analysis of the other article published in *Critical Public Health* that addresses non-human species but that does not reference posthumanism. We selected this text because the only references to posthumanism and public health within our sample were published in *Critical Public Health*. The question we asked when reading this text was: how might posthumanism provide a different theoretical insight? Combining bibliometric analysis with critical discourse analysis in this way allowed us to ask where and how there are synergies between posthumanist theory and public health research.

Findings

The spread of the 7294 articles published in the past 20 years on zoonosis, animals or 'One-health' within the public health literature is unevenly distributed over time (see Supplementary Material, Graph 1). In the first 10 years – between 1995 and 2005 – a small but steady rise is visible. From 2006 onwards, the number of publications per year increases rapidly.

The rise in research regarding zoonosis, animals and/or 'One-health' within the public health literature can be compared with the rise in the general public health literature. Graph 2 (see Supplementary Material) plots the growth of this research and compares it to the growth of the general public health literature. In this graph, the number of publications in 1995 is taken as the baseline. For each year it calculates how much the number of articles has risen in comparison to 1995. For example, a growth of two would mean that the number of publications in that year is double the number of publications in 1995. In Graph 2, we see that the two literatures are increasing at a similar rate from 1995 to 2005. However, research on zoonotic diseases, animals or 'One-health' begins to escalate rapidly relative to the general public health research in 2006. In other words, the research on zoonotic diseases, animals or 'One-health' has become a greater proportion of the total public health research since 2006.

The 7294 publications within the subset of public health, used in this paper, come from 1777 different journals. The top ten journals, in which most articles are published, are shown in Table 2 (see Supplementary Material). Based on the titles of the most occurring journals, it appears that public health research involving non-human animals is primarily applied research that is focused on zoonotic diseases. *Zoonoses and Public Health* publishes the majority of this research by far. Also both the second (*Revue Scientifique et Technique-Office International des Epizooties*) and the tenth journal (*Vector-borne and Zoonotic Diseases*) in our sample focus explicitly on zoonotic diseases. The other journals are either medical (e.g. *Plos One, Epidemiology and Infection, Emerging Infectious Diseases* and *Plos Neglected Tropical Diseases*) or veterinary (e.g. *Veterinary Parasitology, Preventive Veterinary Medicine* and *Veterinary Microbiology*) journals.

To further investigate the content of our sample, and consider where posthumanist critique could contribute, the publications were mapped by means of bibliographic coupling and then divided into clusters. The analysis comprises 6986 of the 7294 documents. Three hundred and eight documents were excluded from the analysis because they were unconnected to any other document (i.e. they either did not share any bibliographic references or there was not any information about the references available). In total, 39 clusters were found, ranging in size from two to 1125 publications. The discussion of the results that follows only addresses the 10 largest clusters, which comprises 72% of the articles in the sample. Table 1 shows the number of publications for the 10 largest clusters in our dataset.

To interpret the clusters, a word analysis of the titles, keywords and abstracts of the articles was executed for each cluster. After removing stop words (such as 'the', 'is', 'at', 'which' and 'on') and punctuation, and transforming all upper case letters to lower case letters, the words were 'stemmed'. This refers to an automated process, which reduces the inflectional forms of a word to a common base form. An example is reducing 'humans' to 'human'. After completing these automated preparations, the frequencies of each word were counted. Since the clusters are homogeneous subsets within the sample, the main topic of the publications in a cluster can be derived by examining the most frequently used words.

The biggest cluster, with 1125 publications, addresses food-borne bacterial infections such as *Salmonella, Escherichia coli* and *Campylobacter jejuni*. The second cluster focuses on nutrition-related public health problems, such as obesity and diabetes. Many of the publications in this cluster used non-human animals as models for human disease. We note this because one of the frequently used words in this cluster is 'model' (mentioned 548 times in this cluster), and was used in specific reference to animal models. The third largest cluster comprises more critical and reflective publications within public health, dealing for instance with policy and health protection programmes. It is within this cluster that a large number of publications can be found that conceptually reflect upon or empirically apply the 'One-health' paradigm. The two publications that explicitly use the terminology of posthumanism can also be found in this cluster (Rock, 2013; Rock et al., 2014).

Clusters four, five and six in Table 1 focus on specific zoonotic diseases: diseases brought forward by helminths such as *Echinococcosis*, vector-borne diseases (for example through ticks or mosquitos) and influenza/viral pandemics (for example avian influenza H5N1). In addition, the final three clusters in Table 1 (clusters eight, nine and ten) also deal with zoonotic diseases. Specifically, these clusters focus on rabies, water-borne parasites (such as *Cryptosporidium* and *Giardia lamblia*) and toxoplasmosis. Finally, the seventh cluster addresses environmental pollution and toxicology. Non-human animals are present in this cluster in two different ways: as experimental models for human diseases and as a site for assessing the exposure of both humans and animals to environmental pollution.

Figure 1 (see Supplementary Material) shows the bibliographic coupling map, in which publications are spatially positioned depending upon the amount of overlap in the references that the publications

Table 1. Overview of clusters with corresponding number of publications.

Cluster	Size
Foodborne infections	1125
Obesity and diabetes	665
One-Health and general	591
Helminths	457
Vector-borne diseases	450
Influenza and viral pandemics	444
Environmental pollution and toxicology	411
Rabies	337
Waterborne parasites	309
Toxoplasmosis	206

cite. Publications positioned close together will have a larger amount of overlap in their bibliographies than publications positioned further away from each other. The colours on the map show the different clusters. The ten main clusters discussed above are marked with the corresponding labels on the map.

On the left hand side, we find the clusters that are focused on zoonotic diseases, or the ways in which human and animal health is interconnected. On the right hand side of the figure, two clusters are found: Environmental pollution and toxicology as well as Obesity and diabetes. These two clusters are spatially rather separate from the other clusters, and differ in content from the other clusters. These two areas of research tend to use animals as models of human disease, or in the case of environmental pollution as co-sufferers. The 'One-health/general' cluster sits right in the middle of our map. This cluster links the public health literature that addresses zoonotic diseases with the research that uses animals as models of human diseases.

Due to the central location of the 'One-health' cluster, we see it as the point of departure for asking if and how posthumanist theory could contribute to public health. 'One-health' is a call for interdisciplinary research and practice regarding the global and interspecies aspects of health and illness in the context of travel as well as declining habitats for non-human, non-domesticated animal species (Craddock & Hinchliffe, 2015; Wolf, 2015); it is embedded in the history of comparative medicine. The most frequently shared references in this cluster (see Supplementary Material, Table 3) gives insight into the key publications within this paradigm and highlight its orientation towards medical science (that includes veterinary medicine). The results presented in Table 3 (see Supplementary Material) are based on a subset of the whole dataset which only includes the 591 publications of cluster 3. From these publications, the most commonly shared publications are listed, which were determined through co-citation analysis. The first column of Supplementary Material Table 3 indicates how many of the 591 publications cite the publication. The first two most frequently cited texts are general public health publications. However, the subsequent publications all focus on the link between human and animal health, and human and animal medicine. The articles were published in medical and veterinary journals in the early years of the 2000s. An exception is the seventh publication, the 1984 book by Calvin Schwabe entitled *Veterinary medicine and human health*. The concept 'one medicine' was coined in this book, which has been further developed and extended into the 'One-health' paradigm in more recent years. We also see from Supplementary Material Table 3 just how important the work of Jakob Zinsstag has been for this cluster, as he is a co-author on three of the ten articles. Further, Zinsstag's work has played a crucial role in raising the importance of Calvin Schwabe's book. The centrality of Schwabe's book could be seen as a critical juncture in the development of One-health, informing its distinctly medical approach today.[1]

Table 4 (see Supplementary Material) shows the publications found within the 'One-health' cluster that have been most cited. We conducted a closer analysis of these articles using critical discourse analysis as these texts have been taken up by other scholars and used in other research programmes the most extensively. These texts are primarily focused on the consequences of non-human agents for human health, such as the species of zoonotic pathogens most likely to be associated with emerging diseases in humans (Taylor, Latham, & Woolhouse, 2001), the factors associated with emerging infectious disease outbreaks in humans (Jones et al., 2008), the problem of antibiotic resistant microbes for human health (Spellberg et al., 2008) and the distribution of ticks and Lyme disease risk (Nicholson & Mather, 1996). One article viewed animals as surrogates for humans in assessing the health effects of chemicals in the environment, in a manner that extends the use of animal models to include animals as sentinels (van der Schalie et al., 1999). The discourse analysis thus mapped onto the bibliometric analysis, wherein One-health links public health research on zoonotic diseases with research using animal models. The former set of articles could be subdivided in terms of focus, where characterizing and classifying pathogens was the goal of some (Cleaveland, Laurenson, & Taylor, 2001; Taylor et al., 2001), understanding the transmission of diseases and its contexts the focus of others (Epstein, 2001; Jones et al., 2008; Mangili & Gendreau, 2005; Nicholson & Mather, 1996), while a third subset of articles were more programmatic or calls to action (Jackson, 2003; Spellberg et al., 2008; Zinsstag, Schelling, Waltner-Toews, & Tanner, 2011).

Non-human species were largely represented as objects for analysis in these texts. There were, however, some instances wherein non-human species were discussed in more agentic terms. For example, microbes were represented as having 'incredible power' that requires 'respect' given their ability to 'inhabit literally every possible climate and environment on the planet' such that 'human beings are nothing more than walking microbial planets' (Spellberg et al., 2008, p. 156). The agency of microbes makes the metaphor of 'war' absurd according to the authors, as it is one that humans could never win. Indeed the authors credit microbes with 'inventing' the primary 'weapon' that humans have in fighting microbes; microbes 'invented' antibiotics over two billion years ago while humans simply 'discovered' antibiotics in the first half of the twentieth century (Spellberg et al., 2008, p. 157). Antimicrobial effectiveness is thus considered a precious resource, one that requires constant stewardship and renewal on the part of humans in order to keep pace with microbial adaptions.

In turn, humans in general and human health specifically were the predominant subjects of these texts. In general, the bifurcation of subjects/objects, culture/nature and human/non-human was implicitly sustained, in a manner that stands in contradiction to posthumanism. However, the animality of humans was nonetheless also at times expressed with statements like: 'Modern society is increasingly aware that humans and culture are components of the natural environment' (Jackson, 2003, p. 191). And the animality of humans presumably makes possible the 'inextricable interconnection of humans, pet animals, livestock and wildlife' that undergirds calls to integrate the medicine and health of humans and animals through One-health (Zinsstag et al., 2011, p. 148). Interestingly, Zinsstag et al. contend that public health has been particularly slow to collaborate and cooperate in addressing zoonotic diseases through a One-health programme because of its focus on human subjects (Zinsstag et al., 2011, p. 151).

To better understand how posthumanism might be integrated into public health research, we looked at the one article in our sample that was published in *Critical Public Health* but that did not use the term posthuman. This article was also located within the 'General/One-Health' cluster.

Mwacalimba's (2012) article in *Critical Public Health* was clustered within the 'One-health' grouping in our analysis. Mwacalimba explored avian influenza preparedness in Zambia. The article does not engage with the term posthuman or any of the posthumanist social theory. It does, however, show the limits of the 'One-health' paradigm by showing how humans and animals are entwined through agriculture and culture. The focus, however, is on understanding how Western concerns regarding avian flu and corresponding international standards overdetermined the preparedness strategies developed in Zambia. This meant that pressing, local human and animal health needs went unaddressed (see also Giles-Vernick, Owona-Ntsama, Landier, & Eyangoh, 2015). Critique here is thus focused on the political economic as opposed to the posthuman. But in the process, the political and economic difficulties associated with integrating human and animal health through the 'One-health' paradigm become increasingly clear. Mwacalimba's article therefore serves as an important lesson for advocates of the 'One-health' paradigm, as avian flu preparedness in Zambia came to be largely controlled by agricultural groups rather than medical or public health groups in a manner that stymied integration. Mwacalimba thus provides an important critique of 'One-health' by following the policy. A posthumanist intervention would ask: what might avian influenza preparedness in Zambia look like by now, following the birds as well?

Discussion

It is interesting to note the rise in public health research involving non-human animals since the 1990s, which from 2006 onwards is even stronger than the rise in the general public health literature. The increased interest in zoonotic diseases accounts for some of the rise in research regarding nonhuman species within public health. High profile zoonotic diseases such as SARS or H1N1 have been a stimulus for this area of research (see also Craddock & Hinchliffe, 2015; Porter, 2015). The heightened concern with zoonotic diseases is exemplified by the change in the name and scope of the *Journal of Veterinary Medicine, Series B* to *Zoonoses and Public Health* in 2007. The focus in this strand of the literature is to understand the pathways through which diseases cross species. But this research agenda also goes beyond nonhuman animals to consider how other-than-animal entities, such as chemicals, also shape human health (see Washburn, 2013 for a discussion). The porosity of individual and species bodies is of key *concern* within this body of research.

The public health literature engages with nonhuman animals in another, distinct way, however. While an extensive part of the literature focuses on zoonotic diseases, public health research also engages in standard biomedical research involving animal models. Biomedical research has long used nonhuman animals as surrogates for humans in research, and public health does this is as well (Friese & Clarke, 2012; Lewis, Atkinson, Harrington, & Featherstone, 2013). The animal model paradigm presumes that species retain certain biological forms and processes through evolution, making it possible for one species to stand as a surrogate for another. This is why Ankeny (2007) argues that comparison is always part of the modelling process, even if it is implicit in the case of 'exemplary' (Bolker, 2009) models. Here the porosity of species bodies is a key *resource* for public health research.

What links these two discrete areas of scholarship is the 'One-health' paradigm. This is clearly demonstrated in Figure 1 (see Supplementary Material), where the 'General/One-health' cluster lies in the middle, between these two literatures in the bibliographic coupling map. The rise in research regarding nonhuman animals in public health is therefore also accounted for by the publication of key articles on the 'One-health' paradigm in the beginning of the 2000s. These articles were frequently cited in later years. As such, the development and further expansion of the 'One-health' literature within the field of public health has boosted the number of publications addressing nonhuman species from the late 2000s onwards. It serves as a link between public health research on zoonotic diseases and public health research that uses animals as models.

The 'One-health' literature is medical in its orientation, and has not engaged with the social sciences (Craddock & Hinchliffe, 2015; Wolf, 2015). This is confirmed in the analysis of the key cited publications within this cluster, which are all published in medical and veterinary journals. From our analysis it can be concluded that the concern with nonhuman animals within public health is based upon the discourse of the 'One-health' paradigm. The critical posthumanist theory from within the social sciences was only present in an extremely limited number of publications. The neglect of the critical posthumanist literature within public health is not surprising, given the concerns of the 'One-health' paradigm and its perceptions of the social sciences. For example, the 'One-health' paradigm has been critiqued for its reliance upon the deficit model, wherein the role of the social sciences is limited to helping to communicate scientific and medical truths to an uninformed public (Craddock & Hinchliffe, 2015).

Conclusion

Interest in nonhuman animals within public health has been informed by the discursive practices of the 'One-health' paradigm, as opposed to the discursive practices of 'posthumanism'. Many of the contributions that Rock et al. (2014) contend posthumanism can make to public health are arguably also already being made by One-health, such as foregrounding: (1) the importance of nonhuman entities for improving human health and subjective well-being (Rock et al., 2014, p. 337; Zinsstag et al., 2011), as evidenced by infectious disease (Jones et al., 2008; Rock et al., 2014, p. 338; Taylor et al., 2001), (2) the use of animals as sentinels (Rock et al., 2014, p. 338; van der Schalie et al., 1999); and (3) the range of nonhuman substances (e.g. microbes, carcinogens) that shape human health (Rock et al., 2014, p. 338; Spellberg et al., 2008). Both posthumanism and One-health also challenge the sharp delineation between physical and social environments (Jackson, 2003; Rock et al., 2014, p. 339).

As such, for posthumanist theory to influence public health research, the differences between 'One-health' and 'posthumanism' needs to be discussed as well. Both posthumanist social theory and 'One-health' emphasize the mutual dependence of humans, other species and other things. But where posthumanist thought is rooted in a philosophical problem, 'One-health' is rooted in an organizational problem. The agency of nonhumans is in turn a focal point and site of potentiality in the more philosophically oriented, posthumanist literature, whereas nonhuman agency is either not considered or considered a problem in the One-health literature. Further, where posthumanism argues that we need to better understand human interactions with other species and things in historically, culturally and politically contingent ways, 'One-health' starts with a biomedical model to argue for a greater integration of human and animal medicine. Finally, and as Green (2012) has pointed out, there is still the assumption of a hierarchy in terms of whose health matters most in the 'One-health' paradigm; it privileges the securitization of human populations in the global North (see also Craddock, 2015; Craddock & Hinchliffe, 2015; Hinchliffe, 2015). The prioritization of certain humans over other humans and other species is contrary to posthumanism. The critical edge of posthumanism could therefore be particularly useful to public health research.

There is a growing social science literature that seeks to critique the 'One-health' paradigm, and these critiques are therefore relevant to current public health research addressing non-human species as well. A recent special issue of *Social Science & Medicine*, for example, critiqued One-health for failing to address power relations (Craddock, 2015; Craddock & Hinchliffe, 2015; Giles-Vernick et al., 2015), which has in turn meant that the social, political and economic embeddedness of human-animal interactions is not addressed by 'One-health' advocates (Coffin, Monje, Asiimwe-Karimu, Amuguni, & Odoch, 2015; Woldehanna & Zimicki, 2015; Wolf, 2015). Posthumanist theory can help public health researchers address these concerns, which are certainly shared by critical public health scholars.

Social scientists have begun to put forward other analytic approaches to the 'One-health' paradigm. This includes cultural anthropology (Wolf, 2015), ethno-ecological history (Giles-Vernick et al., 2015) and participatory epidemiology (Coffin et al., 2015; Paige, Malavé, Mbabazi, Mayer, & Goldberg, 2015). We suggest that posthumanist theories and methods could similarly move forward research concerns with non-human species in public health, particularly critical public health but also more applied public health approaches rooted in social epidemiology.

What would happen if public health research involving non-human animals started with a posthumanist injunction, as opposed to a 'One-health' injunction? If 'One-health' calls for the integration of medical and veterinary expertise, posthumanism would call upon researchers to 'follow the non-human'. Here the non-human agent that is of interest – the animal, the virus, the microbe – is traced as it interacts with humans and other nonhumans. It is a very micro-level approach to seeing how more meso- and macro-level entities, such as networks or structures or meshworks of agency, are produced and/or how diseases are enacted at material and symbolic levels. What would happen if public health research took this up, and began to follow around the nonhuman species of interest and concern for human health? How might that change our analyses? Couldn't public health extend such an approach in the process, by also showing where these relations can be transformed in order to improve the health and wellbeing of humans and other species as well?

Haraway (2008, p. 3) developed her notion of 'becoming with' by asking 'what do I touch when I touch my dog'. Haraway shows that, to answer this question, she needs to tell the natural, social, cultural, political and economic history of her dog's breed through colonialism alongside the natural, social, cultural, political and economic processes shaping her interactions with her dog today. As such, a posthumanist theory that starts with the nonhuman species that is of interest must describe things like local, national and international laws and policies, the history of social relationships between different people and other species and things, the symbolic meaning of nonhuman species within a particular context and the kinds of opportunities and problems these present. But in telling the natural histories of animals or other things as political and economic and cultural and symbolic, the key posthumanist insight could be combined with existing epidemiological practices in a manner that could produce both better knowledge and better policies. As Rock and her colleagues point out, posthumanist approaches are useful to public health because they shift the analysis of infectious diseases from a chain of causation towards a greater understanding of the relationships that drive the incidence of zoonoses (Rock et al., 2014, p. 338). Starting with the nonhuman, tracing its relations and applying critical social theory seems to us to be a necessary next step in public health research involving nonhuman agents.

It is important to emphasize that, while the injunction to 'follow the actor' is more often aligned with actor network theory, we are advocating for a posthumanist approach that is more consistent with Haraway's (1989, 1991, 2008) scholarship then Latour (2005). This is because Haraway uses critical social theory in following nonhuman actors, while Latour does not on the basis of his commitment to a flat ontology. This flat ontology cannot, however, address many of the limitations of the 'One-health' paradigm, as described by the emerging social science literature.[2] We advocate for a posthumanism that engages with history, culture and politics – the stuff of critical public health – in pursuing alternatives to One-health. Such a posthumanist approach has the capacity to both critique and intervene in the processes through which human and nonhuman health alike is 'enacted' (Mol, 2002), in ways that may currently be illness producing.

Notes

1. We would like to thank one of the anonymous reviewers for their comments on this point.
2. That said, Tirado, Gómez, and Rocamora (2015) have analysed influenza using Actor Network Theory and so provide a crucial insight into how the injunction to follow the nonhuman can be put to good use in the context of public health.

Acknowledgements

We would like to thank Sara Cooper and the other organizers of the conference '25 Years of Public Health Criticism: Critique and Nostalgia in Public Health' at the London School of Hygiene and Tropical Medicine for asking us to give a paper on the topic of posthumanism and public health. This conference paper was the basis for this article, and comments at the conference helped tremendously in revising and refining our arguments here. We would also like to thank Angela Cassidy for her comments and suggestions on our handling of One-health in an earlier version of this paper, and Juan Pablo Pardo Guerra for his comments on the bibliometric analysis. The comments from two anonymous reviewers helped us to improve the paper tremendously, for which we are very grateful.

Disclosure statement

No potential conflict of interest was reported by the authors.

References

Ankeny, R. A. (2007). Wormy logic: Model organisms as case-based reasoning. In A N .H. Creager, E. Lunbeck, & M. N. Wise (Eds.), *Science without laws: Model systems, cases, exemplary narratives* (pp. 46–58). Durham, NC: Duke University Press.
Bolker, J. A. (2009). Exemplary and surrogate models: Two modes of representation in biology. *Perspectives in Biology and Medicine, 52*, 485–499.
Cassidy, R., & Mullin, M. (Eds.). (2007). *Where the wild things are now: Domestication reconsidered*. Oxford: Berg.
Cleaveland, S., Laurenson, M. K., & Taylor, L. H. (2001). Diseases of humans and their domestic animals: Pathogen characteristics, host range and the risk of emergence. *Philosophical Transactions for the Royal Society of London B, 356*, 991–999.
Coffin, J. L., Monje, F., Asiimwe-Karimu, G., Amuguni, H. J., & Odoch, T. (2015). A One Health, participatory epidemiology assessment of anthrax (*Bacillus anthracis*) management in Western Uganda. *Social Science & Medicine, 129*, 44–50.
Craddock, S. (2015). Precarious connections: Making therapeutic production happen for malaria and tuberculosis. *Social Science & Medicine, 129*, 36–43.
Craddock, S., & Hinchliffe, S. (2015). Introduction. One world, one health? Social science engagements with the one health agenda. *Social Science & Medicine, 129*, 1–4.
Cubukcu, A. (in press). Thinking against humanity. *London Review of International Law*.
Epstein, P. R. (2001). West Nile virus and the climate. *Journal of Urban Health: Bulletin of the New York Academy of Medicine, 78*, 367–371.
Friese, C., & Clarke, A. E. (2012). Transposing bodies of knowledge and technique: Animal models at work in the reproductive sciences. *Social Studies of Science, 42*, 31–52.
Fukuyama, F. (2002). *Our posthuman future: Consequencs of the biotechnology revolution*. New York, NY: Picador.
Fuller, S. (2011). *Humanity 2.0: What it means to be human past, present and future*. Basingstoke: Palgrave Macmillan.
Giles-Vernick, T., Owona-Ntsama, J., Landier, J., & Eyangoh, S. (2015). The puzzle of Buruli ulcer transmission, ethno-ecological history and the end of 'love' in the Akonolinga district, Cameroon. *Social Science & Medicine, 129*, 20–27.
Green, J. (2012). 'One health, one medicine' and critical public health. *Critical Public Health, 22*, 377–381.
Habermas, J. (2003). *The Future of Human Nature*. Cambridge: Polity.
Haraway, D. J. (1989). *Primate visions: Gender, race, and nature in the world of modern science*. New York: Routledge.

Haraway, D. J. (1991). A cyborg manifesto: science, technology, and socialist-feminism in the late twentieth century. In *Simians, cyborgs, and women: the reinvention of nature* (pp. 149–182). New York, NY: Routledge.

Haraway, D. J. (2008). *When species meet*. Minneapolis: Minnesota University Press.

Hinchliffe, S. (2015). More than one world, more than one health: Re-configuring interspecies health. *Social Science & Medicine, 129*, 28–35.

Ingold, T. (2011). *Being alive: Essays on movement, knowledge and description*. London: Routledge.

Jackson, L. E. (2003). The relationship of urban design to human health and condition. *Landscape and Urban Planning, 64*, 191–200.

Jager, S., & Maier, F. (2009). Theoretical and methodological aspects of foucauldian critical discourse analysis and dispositive analysis. In R. Wodak & M. Meyer (Eds.), *Methods of critical discourse analysis* (2nd ed., pp. 34–63). London: Sage.

Jarneving, B. (2007). Bibliographic coupling and its application to research-front and other core documents. *Journal of Informetrics, 1*, 287–307.

Jones, K. E., Patel, N. G., Levy, M. A., Storeygard, A., Balk, D., Gittleman, J. L., & Daszak, P. (2008). Global trends in emerging infectious diseases. *Nature, 451*, 990–994.

Latour, B. (2005). *Reassembling the social: An introduction to actor-network-theory*. Oxford: Oxford University Press.

Leach, H. M. (2003). Human domestication reconsidered. *Current Anthropology, 44*, 349–368.

Lewis, J., Atkinson, P., Harrington, J., & Featherstone, K. (2013). Representation and practical accomplishment in the laboratory: when is an animal model good-enough? *Sociology, 47*, 776–792.

Mangili, A., & Gendreau, M. A. (2005). Transmission of infectious diseases during commercial air travel. *The Lancet, 365*, 989–996.

Mol, A. (2002). *The body multiple: Ontology in medical practice*. Durham, NC: Duke University.

Mwacalimba, K. K. (2012). Globalised disease control and response distortion: A case study of avian influenza pandemic preparedness in Zambia. *Critical Public Health, 22*, 391–405.

Nicholson, M. C., & Mather, T. N. (1996). Methods for evaluating lyme disease risks using geographic information systems and geospatial analysis. *Entomological Society of America, 33*, 711–720.

Paige, S. B., Malavé, C., Mbabazi, E., Mayer, J., & Goldberg, T. L. (2015). Uncovering zoonoses awareness in an emeging disease 'hotspot'. *Social Science & Medicine, 129*, 78–86.

Porter, N. H. (2016). Ferreting things out: Biosecurity, pandemic flue and the transformation of experimental systems. *BioSocieties, 11*, 22–45.

Rock, M. J. (2013). Pet bylaws and posthumanist health promotion: A case study of urban policy. *Critical Public Health, 23*, 201–212.

Rock, M. J., Degeling, C., & Blue, G. (2014). Toward stronger theory in critical public health: Insights from debates surrounding posthumanism. *Critical Public Health, 24*, 337–348.

Savulescu, J., & Bostrom, N. (Eds.). (2009). *Human enhancement*. Oxford: Oxford University Press.

Spellberg, B., Guidos, R., Gilbert, D., Bradley, J., Boucher, H. W., Scheld, W. M., & … Edwards, J. J. (2008). The epidemic of antibiotic-resistant infections: A call to action for the medical community from the infectious diseases society of america. *Clinical Infectious Diseases, 46*, 155–164.

Taylor, L. H., Latham, S. M., & Woolhouse, M. E. J. (2001). Risk factors for human disease emergence. *Philosophical Transactions for the Royal Society of London B, 356*, 983–989.

Tirado, F., Gómez, A., & Rocamora, V. (2015). The global condition of epidemics: Panoramas in A (H1N1) influenza and their consequences for One World One Health programme. *Social Science & Medicine, 129*, 113–122.

van der Schalie, W. H., Gardner, H. S. J., Bantle, J. A., De Rosa, C. T., Finch, R. A., Reif, J S, & … Stokes, W. S. (1999). Animals as sentinels of human health hazards of environmental chemicals. *Environmental Health Perspectives, 107*, 309–315.

van Eck, N. J., Waltman, L., Dekker, R., & van den Berg, J. (2010). A comparison of two techniques for bibliometric mapping: Multidimensional scaling and VOS. *Journal of the American Society for Information Science and Technology, 61*, 2405–2416.

Waltman, L., van Eck, N. J., & Noyons, E. C. (2010). A unified approach to mapping and clustering of bibliometric networks. *Journal of Informetrics, 4*, 629–635.

Washburn, R. (2013). The social significance of human biomonitoring. *Sociology Compass, 7*, 162–179.

Wodak, R., & Meyer, M. (2009). Critical discourse analysis: History, agenda, theory and methodology. In R. Wodak & M. Meyer (Eds.), *Methods of critical discourse analysis* (2nd ed., pp. 1–33). London: Sage.

Woldehanna, S., & Zimicki, S. (2015). An expanded One Health model: Integrating social science and One Health to inform study of human-animal interface. *Social Science & Medicine, 129*, 87–95.

Wolf, M. (2015). Is there really such a thing as 'one health'? Thinking about a more than human world from the perspective of cultural anthropology. *Social Science & Medicine, 129*, 5–11.

Wolfe, C. (2010). *What is posthumanism?*. Minneapolis: Minnesota University Press.

Zinsstag, J., Schelling, E., Waltner-Toews, D., & Tanner, M. (2011). From 'one medicine' to 'one health' and systemic approachs to health and well-being. *Preventive Veterinary Medicine, 101*, 148–156.

Who or what is 'the public' in critical public health? Reflections on posthumanism and anthropological engagements with One Health

Melanie J. Rock

ABSTRACT

This paper extends the terms of engagement between social science, posthumanist debates and One Health by questioning whether 'the public' may include non-human animals. The One Health concept refers to interdependence between human beings and non-human species in socio-ecological systems. One Health interventions and critiques have tended to emphasize the prevention of zoonotic infections, whereas this paper reflects on more than a decade of engaged research in One Health promotion. Repeatedly, this particular approach to One Health promotion has highlighted the imprint of multi-species entanglements in public life, especially the problematization and politicization of people's pets. Serious consideration for multi-species entanglements cautions against conflating 'the public' with human beings and human interests, to the exclusion of all others. Human beings have never lived separate and apart from non-human species, and we all depend on shared environments. To do justice to multi-species entanglements, socio-ecological theory should undergo expansion in health promotion.

Introduction

'I am not a posthumanist', Haraway (2008, 19) has declared. Somewhat ironically, she makes this statement in the inaugural volume of a book series titled 'Posthumanities'. The broader context for this statement includes the fact that Haraway does not want to be regarded as a post-feminist. Moreover, she was calling upon critical theorists to pay more attention to myriad ways in which human beings are linked to one another and to non-human life, and to recognize injustice amidst such linkages. Overall, Haraway (2008, pp. 134, 135) argues that any instance of human flourishing is inevitably multi-species in nature. Following on from her disavowal of the 'posthumanist' identity, Haraway (2008, p. 19) stated, 'I am who I become with companion species, who and which make a mess of categories in the making of kin and kind'.

Also in the 'Posthumanities' book series, but in a later volume, Wolfe (Wolfe, 2010, p. xv) wrote, 'Posthumanism names an historical moment in which the decentring of the human by its imbrication in technical, medical, informatics, and economic networks is increasingly impossible to ignore'. I subscribe to this definition of posthumanism. At the same time, I am sympathetic to Haraway's concern about the potential for fashionable trends in critical theory to obscure inequity. Unlike others who have written about social-*qua*-environmental justice in health promotion (Frohlich & Abel, 2014; Masuda, Poland, & Baxter, 2010; Rydin et al., 2012; Shortt, Rind, Pearce, & Mitchell, 2014; Taylor, Floyd, Whitt-Glover, & Brooks, 2007), however, I take multi-species entanglements to be central.

For anthropologists, myself included, Haraway's (2008, p. 19) reference to 'the making of kin and kind' has particular resonance. Our discipline is undergirded by the notion of a human species that is distinct from – yet distantly related to – all other animals. Accordingly, 'an "anthropocentric" focus is something to be expected from *anthro*pologists'. (Hurn, 2010, p. 27; emphasis in original). Notwithstanding the discipline's humanist foundations, anthropologists' fieldwork has repeatedly challenged anthropocentrism. Over the last decade, interest in human-animal studies and anthrozoology (i.e. the study of humans' interactions with members of non-human species) grew exponentially within both physical anthropology and sociocultural anthropology (Fuentes, 2012; Smart, 2014). Related concerns have begun to influence medical anthropology and public health. To name but one example, Nading (2014) reports on ethnographic research as a medical anthropologist alongside Nicaraguan community health workers, as they investigated cases of and risks for dengue fever. This infection is mosquito-borne, yet its incidence in urban Nicaragua is driven by inequity on local and global scales.

Previously, Nading (2013) published an exemplary literature review, titled 'Humans, animals and health: From ecology to entanglement'. Therein, he aligned with Haraway's (2008, p. 513) contention that interactions amongst human and non-human beings arise from 'the material-semiotic requirements of getting on together in specific lifeworlds'. Nading (2013) argues that human health depends on non-human species as well as on environments, but not as discrete things. Indeed, Nading (2013, p. 61) contends that 'multi-species entanglements' are germane to 'the production of life itself', and thus to health. This paper extends the principles of health promotion to consider multi-species entanglements and the concept of One Health.

For the purposes of this paper, One Health refers to interdependence between human and non-human beings in complex socio-ecological systems (Zinsstag, Schelling, Waltner-Toews, & Tanner, 2011). Unlike prevailing socio-ecological theory in health promotion (Richard, Gauvin, & Raine, 2011), the concept of One Health emphasizes multi-species interactions and how these interactions are situated. Notwithstanding the relevance of the social sciences to the study of socio-ecological systems, engagement of critical social scientists with the One Health concept and its applications remains incipient (Craddock & Hinchliffe, 2015; Green, 2012). Thus far, One Health applications – and corresponding critiques – have mainly focused on preventing the spread of zoonoses. Below, by contrast, I focus on the potential for One Health promotion via human-dog interactions within urbanized environments.

Whereas the One Health concept crystallized about ten years ago (Zinsstag et al., 2011), social scientists and veterinarians have sought to enhance emotional connections between people and dogs over the course of nearly four decades, As Haraway (2008) observes, 'In the United States, dogs became "companion animals" both in contrast and in addition to "pets" and "working and sporting dogs," around the late 1970s in the context of social scientific investigations of animals such as dogs to human health and wellbeing'. Hereafter in this paper, I use the terms 'pet' and 'companion animal' interchangeably. Nevertheless, the term 'companion animal' might suggest a stronger human-animal bond as well as higher socio-economic status than the term 'pet'. Also, some who use the term 'companion animal' object to classifying any animal as property, whereas my own position is that the legal status of property is not inherently injurious to non-human animals (Rock & Degeling, 2013).

As a social movement, animal welfare is international in scope, as illustrated by the legal legitimacy of 'street dogs' as a public presence in cities throughout India (Srinivasan, 2013). Even in such disadvantaged environments as the city of N'Djaména in Chad, people may single out particular 'street dogs' for attention, by feeding them and bringing them to be vaccinated against rabies (Durr et al., 2009). Meanwhile, approximately 25% to 50% of all households in Western countries include dogs (Christian et al., 2016). In addition, caring for dogs as household pets has recently become popular in some non-Western cities, notably in China and Japan (Hansen, 2013; Headey, Na, & Zheng, 2007; Shibata et al., 2012).

The history of how so many urban-dwelling dogs came to live within households as pets reflects how social reformers engaged with rabies control in the nineteenth century (Grier, 2006; Pemberton &

Worboys, 2013). Dog-owners in urban areas, especially upper-class women, objected to decrees that all pet dogs should be muzzled whenever in public, and they proposed instead to walk their canine companions on leashes (Howell, 2012). Hence, dog-ownership and dog-walking are germane to a critical perspective on the history of public health, as well as to health promotion in contemporary times. Dog-walking in cities still involves some risks, notably the potential for dogs to intimidate, to attack and to spread infections (Smith, Semeniuk, Rock, & Massolo, 2015; Toohey & Rock, 2011; Westgarth et al., 2009). Nevertheless, dog-walking also can support physical, mental and social well-being, for both the human and canine participants (Westgarth, Christley, & Christian, 2014). Some people without dogs of their own may also benefit from regular dog-walking, for example, when dog-walkers and the dogs themselves informally patrol neighbourhoods (Toohey & Rock, 2011). A key question for health promotion, therefore, ought to be how to maximize the benefits of human-dog companionship in urban environments, while simultaneously minimizing associated risks.

A decade of engaged research in One Health promotion, focusing mainly on dog-ownership and dog-walking, has led me to pose the question, 'Who or what is "the public" in critical public health?' I pose this question because I have become uneasy with the extent to which conceptualizations of 'the public' remain tethered to anthropocentrism. For example, *public anthropologists* seek 'to redress *human problems* associated with inequities and injustices' (Maida & Beck, 2015, p. 3; emphasis added), including the uneven distribution of sickness in human populations. Many medical anthropologists have, accordingly, treated human sicknesses as the epitome of human problems, without much concern for distinguishing public anthropology from public health. For the medical anthropologist Marsland (2014, p. 75), however, any worthwhile 'ethnographic understanding of public health includes a clarification of what the "public" means'. With respect to the public health officials who featured in her fieldwork, Marsland (2014, p. 75) contends that the notion of 'a public as a critical rational debating group does not exist'. Rather, these officials 'imagine something akin to a crowd or a population, which are quite different things', she maintains, 'than a public (Marsland, 2014, p. 76). 'Publics have reason and are bound together by their minds, whereas populations are ideally composed of masses of ordered bodies' and crowds are 'unreasonable, unruly, and even dangerous' (Marsland, 2014, p. 85). Here, Marsland leans on the dominant way of thinking about publics in the social sciences, which emphasizes rational discourse as a higher-order trait in human beings (Warner, 2002).

Meanwhile, 'public health' is often understood by insiders as 'the efforts organized by society to protect, promote, and restore the people's health' (Last, 2001, 145). Such a definition implies that 'the public' is synonymous with 'the population as a whole' (Last, 2001, p. 145). Krieger (2012), however, contends that the 'population' concept is unacceptably ambiguous in public health. Accordingly, she calls for scholars aligned with public health 'to expand and deepen their theorizing about who and what makes populations' (Krieger, 2012, p. 649). She also asserts that human populations comprise 'relational beings' (Krieger, 2012, p. 649). Krieger's arguments might apply equally to 'the public' in public health. As a field, critical public health must pay more heed to the conceptualization of 'public'. Furthermore, the 'relational beings' (Krieger, 2012, p. 649) germane to public health are not all human in nature. For instance, the 'relational beings' relevant to public health include dogs. Below, I discuss the place of dogs in family, community and public life. With the City of Calgary, Alberta, Canada serving as a case-study, I reflect on the implications of multi-species entanglements for critical public health as a field.

Setting and methodology

All of the examples cited in this paper come from a series of externally funded projects in the City of Calgary, and the University of Calgary's Conjoint Health Research Ethics Board approved and monitored each of these projects. The data-set includes interview transcripts, fieldnotes, questionnaires and policy documents. Ethnographically speaking, however, much of my One Health research has been 'informal' (Agar, 2006; Katz, 2006). By 'informal' I mean that insights have arisen from day-to-day immersion in social life, casual encounters in places like parks, meetings with City officials, and events involving charitable organizations and public health agencies. These insights have been refined through 'formal' research projects.

The City of Calgary is a sprawling city located about 100 km from the Rocky Mountains. This territory traditionally belongs to the people of the Treaty 7 region in Southern Alberta. The City of Calgary is also home to the Metis Nation of Alberta, Region 3. More than 1.3 million people now live in Calgary, alongside more than 120,000 dogs and upwards of 100,000 cats kept for companionship (Rock, 2013). As the City has grown in recent decades, the human population has become more diverse, but at the same time, inequitable in terms of socio-economic measures such as education, home-ownership and income (Smart, 2001; Tanasescu, Wing-tak, & Smart, 2010). Nationally and internationally, Calgary has a reputation for being 'pet-friendly', and this reputation encompasses collaborative relationships with animal welfare organizations and public engagement with respect to policies that aim to shape human-animal interactions in daily life (Rock, 2013; Rock et al., 2016a).

From diabetes in multi-species families to dog-walking

More than a decade prior to the current interest in the 'three-minute thesis', I had learned to truncate my response to the question, 'What are you studying for your PhD?' into a single word: diabetes. Uttering that word, 'diabetes', typically sparked a story about my interlocutor's own health, or about a relative, and sometimes discussion about the challenges faced by children living with type 1 diabetes or by Indigenous people living with type 2 diabetes. Yet, on more than one occasion, people talked about dogs and cats living with diabetes. Sometimes they told stories about their own pets; other times, they talked about a pet belonging to a friend or a neighbour. Nothing in my training, background reading or doctoral fieldwork in medical anthropology had primed me to anticipate that pets would exemplify life with diabetes for many people. In fact, I recalled that dogs procured from the City of Toronto had served as animal models in the experimental research that led to insulin therapy (Bliss, 1982/2000). Hence, the social phenomenon of dogs and cats being treated daily with insulin, as patients in their own right, came as a surprise. I was curious enough to write a grant so that I could investigate further, and I was fortunate enough to receive funding for ethnographic research on the topic of diabetic pet-care (Rock & Babinec, 2008, 2010).

In telling stories about diabetic pet-care, dog-owners often described dog-walking as a way of taking care of their dogs as well as themselves. Still, canine diabetes could interrupt or reshape dog-walking routines. For example, one middle-aged man recalled:

> I had him [his dog] crash on me a couple of times where his blood sugar went so low that he became very disoriented and couldn't walk. One time I had to carry him about seven, eight blocks home, and after that I started carrying something with glucose in it in case that ever happened again, I wasn't carrying him home. (Rock & Babinec, 2008, 336)

Just as I was collecting stories like this one, about dog-walking as a facet of caring for a diabetic dog, researchers concerned with promoting physical activity began to take dog-walking seriously (Cutt, Giles-Corti, Knuiman, & Burke, 2007). This confluence of interests led into a series of studies to examine dog-walking as a sociocultural practice that is broadly relevant to health promotion.

In one of these subsequent studies of dog-walking, an older man admitted that he had become less active since the death of his family's dog. He explained in an interview,

> It was not just a walking experience, it was a … it was a total, an all-in experience … So the dog might get out of bed and get you going in the morning, and you enjoyed it all the way through. (Degeling & Rock, 2013, 401)

Towards the end of this dog's life, their dog-walking routine ceased to include a neighbourhood park where the two of them had been regular visitors for years (Degeling & Rock, 2013, p. 403). Parks are key assets for dog-walking (McCormack, Rock, Toohey, & Hignell, 2010; Westgarth et al., 2014). More generally, urban parks can serve as salutogenic settings, so they are important for environmental justice (Frohlich & Abel, 2014; Frohlich & Potvin, 1999; Masuda et al., 2010; Taylor et al., 2007).

The dog-walker quoted above was drawn from a pool of Calgarians who had previously completed a telephone interview and a self-administered questionnaire regarding physical activity. Overall, the dog-owners were three times more likely than were the non-dog-owners to walk regularly for recreation year-round within their neighbourhoods (Lail, McCormack, & Rock, 2011). This finding is all the more remarkable considering that winters can be harsh in Calgary. Also, 'walkability' in Calgary tends to be sub-optimal, according to standard measures (McCormack, Shiell, Doyle-Baker, Friedenreich, & Sandalack, 2014). Furthermore, we found that amongst the dog-owners who were 50-plus in age, frequent dog-walking corresponded with feeling a sense of community (Toohey, McCormack, Doyle-Baker, Adams, & Rock, 2013). In sum, caring for a dog may protect against some of the negative impacts on physical, mental and social well-being that public health researchers have repeatedly linked with weather conditions and built environments (McCormack et al., 2014).

Nevertheless, dog-walking is not always a feasible or a positive experience for dog-owners, even in this 'pet-friendly' city. As reported by a mother of two school-aged children in an extended interview,

> I never took the dog to school because they don't like having the dogs around the school … I know they had issue with some people always bringing their dogs and the dogs would bark at the fence. You know? And I just thought, you know, I don't want to do that. (Degeling & Rock, 2013, 403)

According to local policy, dogs are not allowed in schoolyards (Rock, 2013). Yet in this participant's neighbourhood, sociocultural norms extended the no-dogs-allowed prohibition to public property, including sidewalks, where leashed dogs are officially allowed. Consequently, the participant typically drove her children to school in a privately owned vehicle, rather than dog-walking alongside them on weekday mornings. On the one hand, the mother's decision to keep the family dog away from her children's schoolyard could be viewed as respectful. On the other hand, driving rather than walking each morning to school could be seen as a lost opportunity for physical activity for families.

In other households, dog-walking routines explicitly took an individual dog's temperament into account. For example, one dog-owner explained that she employed a professional dog-walker to help manage her dog's separation anxiety (Degeling & Rock, 2013, p. 403). In this case, caring for the dog translated into dog-walking for someone outside the household, in addition to the dog-walking that was undertaken by human members of the family. Another participant explained that she employed a professional dog-walker, not to treat mental illness in her dog as in the previous example, but to cope with traits that she attributed to 'breed'. Still, she made allowance for differences in canine personalities:

> It's very hard to walk three hunting dogs at the same time. So that's why they get runs, as opposed to regular walks … They're really nice dogs, and they're not stupid … William is a strong dog; he alone is a handful. (Degeling & Rock, 2013, 403)

Consideration of 'breed' with respect to other people's dogs also carried into public space. For example, a different dog-owner stated,

> I'm very, very wary of Pitbulls if they're ever off a leash … I will call out a long way ahead to find out if that's a friendly dog, because I've had bad experiences with Pitbulls. (Degeling & Rock, 2013, 403)

The City of Calgary neither has restrictions on owning Pitbull-type dogs, nor on bringing such dogs to off-leash areas in City parks. Indeed, Calgary has never had what is known as 'breed-specific legislation' (BSL) on the books. Upon overhauling its policy framework on pets in 2006, the City explicitly rejected BSL as a measure to protect public health and safety. Rather, officers investigate each dog-aggression complaint, and following serious dog-bites, the City may deem a dog to be a 'Vicious Animal'. Amongst other restrictions, 'Vicious Animals' are banned from designated off-leash areas in parks (City of Calgary 2006/2016). To meet the criteria for a 'Vicious Animal', a dog's victims may be human or non-human.

Rather than adopting and enforcing BSL, the City has earned an international reputation (e.g. Parliament of Victoria, 2016) for developing and implementing a policy framework that regards people and pets as elements that co-exist within cities, as complex socio-ecological systems. More specifically, this framework emphasizes improvements that could accrue from simultaneously: (1) preventing threats and nuisances from pets; (2) licensing pets with the City and identifying them with collar-tags, microchips or both; (3) providing veterinary services for pets, notably sterilization surgeries; (4) procuring pets ethically; and (5) meeting the emotional and physical needs of pets (Rock, Adams, Degeling, Massolo, & McCormack, 2015). Moreover, [Calgary]'s policy framework portrays people, pets and wildlife as actors and as in a posthumanist approach to health promotion (Rock, 2013). In parallel, City parks have been construed as ecological resources that need to be protected from overuse by people and their canine companions (Toohey & Rock, 2015). Below, I elaborate on the implications of this posthumanist approach to One Health promotion with reference to the City of Calgary's current policy on off-leash dogs. This policy example raises intriguing questions about the nature and orientation of critical public health.

From dog-walking to multi-species communities and publics

In the decade since the City of Calgary reformed its policy framework on pets, off-leash dogs have been its most vexing pet-related policy issue. Importantly, given the lack of BSL in this jurisdiction, dog-bites in parks where the City allows dogs to be off-leash have not been a major concern (Toohey & Rock, 2015). Unlike 'dog parks' in many cities, especially in the United States (Matisoff & Noonan, 2012), off-leash areas in Calgary tend to be unfenced and in principle, they are open to dog-walkers, supervised dogs, and non-dog-walkers (Rock, Graham, Massolo, & McCormack, 2016b). Some off-leash areas sit within neighbourhood parks, whereas others comprise vast spaces nested within natural grasslands and brush. In 2011, when City Council revised its previous off-leash policy and proposed to increase its off-leash inventory, more than 17% of the City's parkland had already been designated for off-leash access (Rock et al., 2016a).

A key change in Calgary's revised off-leash policy was to allow dog-walkers who lived outside of the residential neighbourhood containing as a given park to participate in decision-making (Rock et al., 2016a). Under the previous policy, only paid-up members of a neighbourhood association recognized by the City could vote on proposals concerning off-leash areas in nearby parks. And to vote, residents had to attend their neighbourhood association's annual general meeting in person. Dog-walkers successfully pressed the point in the local media and with City officials that they could become bona fide stakeholders for parks beyond the boundaries of their residential neighbourhoods, in the course of regularly bringing their dogs to these places (Toohey & Rock, 2015). And in response to pressure from dog-walking communities, the City has explicitly acknowledged that allowing dogs to be off-leash in public space can be beneficial to the physical, mental and social well-being of dog-owners. As stated in its current policy on off-leash dogs in parks,

> Along with traditionally recognized and high-demand recreation activities, there is recognition that walking/exercising with your dog off-leash is a valid form of recreational activity. (City of Calgary, 2011, p. 9)

In other words, [Calgary]'s current policies on off-leash dogs recognize that dog-walking is not strictly a matter of individual responsibility vested in dog-owners (Toohey & Rock, 2015).

With time, I came to conclude that dog-walking communities are multi-species in nature. The notion of multi-species communities is somewhat at odds with foundational knowledge in health promotion, which is anthropocentric when it comes to social relationships within ecological systems. For instance, the World Health Organization (WHO) Health Promotion Glossary defines 'community' as follows:

> A specific group of *people*, often living in a defined geographical area, who share a common *culture, values and norms*, are arranged in a social structure according to relationships which the community has developed over a period of time. Members of a community gain their personal and social identity by sharing common beliefs, values and norms which have been developed by the community in the past and may be modified in the future. They exhibit some *awareness* of their identity as a group, and share common needs and a commitment to meeting them. (Nutbeam, 1998, 353–354, emphasis added)

Notwithstanding a tendency in health promotion to emphasize geographically based communities (Petersen, 1996), the WHO acknowledges that people may belong to 'a range of communities based on variables such as geography, occupation, social and leisure interests' (Nutbeam, 1998, p. 354).

Dog-walking certainly is a common leisure activity, notably in urban parks, through which people establish relationships with one another and may share a 'common culture, values and norms' (Nutbeam, 1998, p. 353). In the Australian city of Perth, for instance, researchers found that dog-ownership and dog-walking created 'ripple effects' that enhanced community capacity, trust and overall well-being (Wood, Giles-Corti, & Bulsara, 2005; Wood, Giles-Corti, Bulsara, & Bosch, 2007). These researchers, however, stopped short of claiming that dogs were full-fledged members of the communities in question. Yet my team's research, together with posthumanist theory, points in just that direction. In sharing my team's research on dog-walking and off-leash policy, I have found that staking a claim about multi-species communities is provocative, although less so than claiming that a given public may combine human and non-human members.

In other words, I am claiming that in places like off-leash parks, interactions between people and dogs, amongst people, *and* amongst dogs give rise to social structures that are multi-species in composition. Therefore, to the extent that the people enfolded within a dog-walking community do share 'a common culture, values and norms' (Nutbeam, 1998, p. 353), then dogs are inextricably part of the mix. These pets may 'exhibit some awareness of their identity as a group' (Nutbeam, 1998, p. 354), for example, by seeking out familiar humans and dogs upon arrival at a park. Furthermore, the 'common needs' (Nutbeam, 1998, p. 354), that dog-walkers strive to meet may be hybrids of human and canine interests. Certainly that was the case as dog-walkers repeatedly rallied to shore up and then to expand [Blinded-City]'s off-leash park inventory (Rock et al., 2016a; Toohey & Rock, 2015). Dog-walking communities instigated the creation of multi-species publics, first at the scale of the City as a whole, and then in relation to specific parks and surrounding neighbourhoods.

Dogs were not only instrumental to establishing off-leash access as a policy issue for the City of Calgary, but dogs participated (albeit indirectly) in the reform of a health-related policy as bona fide members in multi-species publics. Yet to make such a claim, about dogs as political actors, may seem counter-intuitive. If indeed 'public health' consists of the 'the efforts organized by society to protect, promote, and restore the people's health' (Last, 2001, p. 145), then those of us aligned to critical public health ought to question the composition of 'society;' how 'efforts [are] organized;' and the differential impacts arising from such efforts, not only amongst people, but also on non-human animals and on ecosystems. Put another way, engagements with One Health are thoroughly relevant to critical public health, and Calgary is simply a microcosm for a global situation.

Amongst critical theorists, conceptualizations of 'the public' are closely associated with rational discourse that is, at least in principle, transparent and open to everyone (Warner, 2002). Yet, in contradistinction to this discursive tradition, there also exists a materialist tradition in the study of public affairs. The materialist tradition is closely associated with the philosophy of pragmatism, especially the contributions of Dewey (1927/1991), who famously argued that publics emerge when existing arrangements cannot resolve human problems. For Dewey, there is no such thing as 'the public'. Rather, Dewey's scholarship implies that multiple publics co-exist and may displace one another.

In what might be described as a posthumanist interpretation of Dewey (1927/1991), Marres (2007) contends that human problems cannot be understood accurately without taking non-humans into account. That is because non-human entities are integral to the formation of problems, and non-human entities are essential to the application of remedies (see also Marres & Lezaun, 2011). In arguing that publics invariably include non-human elements, Marres (2010, 2016) has called attention to communication infrastructure and mundane objects, such as teapots. Marres has not gone so far as to argue that publics may enfold non-human animals as constituents.

Nonetheless, integrating insights from Haraway, amongst other theorists, opens up the possibility of multi-species publics (Blue, 2015; Blue & Rock, 2014; Instone & Sweeney, 2014). Based on their examination of multiple dog-related tensions in Australian cities, Instone and Sweeney (2014, p. 784) conclude that 'publics' need to be redefined 'as a more-than-human arena of complex and multiple relations'. As a medical anthropologist aligned to critical public health, I could not agree more.

With respect to the City of Calgary's policy review regarding off-leash dogs, disparate views on and interactions with non-human animals were, inherently and inextricably, at issue (Toohey & Rock, 2015). Additional non-humans of interest, in relation to the identification of problems and potential solutions, included leashes, collars, park signage, dog-feces, waste disposal units, city streets, privately owned vehicles, parking lots, public parks and mechanisms for inscribing the views of citizens (Rock et al., 2016a). The City sought to balance the mixed views of dog-owners and non-dog-owners; to reach consensus whenever possible; and when consensus could not be found, to make principled decisions that could withstand scrutiny. Despite the efforts that were made, fairness proved difficult to achieve in practice (Rock et al., 2016a).

As with human beings, to be politically influential, companion animals require representation. And as illustrated by the case of Calgary's off-leash policy, dogs have managed to acquire political influence through their complex and evolving relationships with one another and with human beings in urban areas. By way of example, off-leash dogs became a policy issue for the City largely in relation to controversy that began within a particular park and then spilled over into media coverage. This park is located in a gentrifying neighbourhood whose establishment dates from the late 1950s. The City already allowed off-leash dogs in this park, which was fenced on three sides, when the neighbourhood association asked the City to install fencing and a gate on the fourth side, so as to fully enclose the park. Enclosing the park could prevent the dogs from escaping and thus protect them from automobile traffic. Shortly thereafter, dogs and people from outside the immediate neighbourhood poured into the park and nearby side-streets. One reason for the sudden surge in visits was that a dog-walking interest group shared the news via social media that a large fully fenced park with an off-leash designation was now publicly accessible. Many local residents objected to the new 'crowd', to use terminology employed by Marsland (2014) to refer to unruly groups. Tactics employed by disgruntled residents to regain control over 'their neighbourhood' included lodging formal complaints with the City, speaking with elected officials, and consenting to be interviewed by journalists (Toohey & Rock, 2015).

Holmberg (2013) has also referred to dogs and people as 'a trans-species urban crowd' in the relation to off-leash politics, but in another location. As my team has done with respect to the City of Calgary, Holmberg (2013) analysed a series of efforts to convert off-leash controversy into political gains, especially claims over territory. I infer that what began as dog-walking communities became 'a trans-species urban crowd' (Holmberg, 2013) and then a multi-species public. Furthermore, multi-species publics appear to have taken shape elsewhere in relation to on-leash and off-leash policies (Holmberg, 2013; Instone & Sweeney, 2014; Urbanik & Morgan, 2013; Walsh, 2011). Rather than conceiving of any and all publics as being bound together first and foremost by rational thought (Marsland, 2014; Warner, 2002), multi-species entanglements undergird the publics that have formed in relation to on-leash and off-leash policies.

Conclusions

This paper has interrogated the meaning of 'the public' in critical public health, with reference to anthropological theory, debates surrounding posthumanism, and an ethnographic research programme in the realm of One Health promotion. Institutionally speaking, public health has long acknowledged non-human species along with shared environments, yet mainly through an emphasis on human mastery. By way of illustration, the Ottawa Charter for Health Promotion states that 'a stable eco-system' is a pre-requisite for human health (WHO, 1986). More recently, a high-profile article on 'healthy cities' as complex systems only acknowledged non-human animals as vermin (Rydin et al., 2012).

Recent critiques have called for health promoters involved in the 'healthy cities' movement to engage more fulsomely with environmental politics (Masuda et al., 2010; Patrick, Dooris, & Poland, 2016), and this paper extends the argument about sharpening socio-ecological thinking in health promotion and the 'healthy cities' movement. More specifically, this paper calls attention to people's pets as both agents and vectors of social change in urbanized environments. Pets do not count as full-fledged citizens, but they do belong to urban families and communities, and they are constituents in urban publics. Not only do urban policies influence non-human lives, but sometimes non-human animals figure amongst the intended beneficiaries, as illustrated by the existence of parks where off-leash dogs are allowed.

Most One Health interventions, evaluations and critiques have emphasized quests for control over zoonotic infections (Blue & Rock, 2011; Craddock & Hinchliffe, 2015; Green, 2012). Nevertheless, the conceptual basis of One Health resonates with Haraway's (2008) argument that flourishing is, inevitably, a multi-species endeavour (Rock & Degeling, 2015, 2016). Health promotion, therefore, pertains not only to human well-being, but also to non-human animals and their well-being. Somewhat counter-intuitively, therefore, I am led to conclude that many issues in a 'health in all policies' approach to health promotion entail the formation of multi-species communities and publics.

Acknowledgements

I presented an earlier version as a CIHR/IPPH Visiting Lecturer (ICT-138,054) when the University of Sussex hosted a joint conference of the European Association for Social Anthropology's Medical Anthropology Network and the Royal Anthropological Institute's Medical Anthropology Committee. More specifically, I presented at the University of Sussex in a panel convened by Simon Cohn and Rebecca Lynch on posthumanism, medical anthropology and global health. I gratefully acknowledge insights that were shared with me by the research participants and within my research team (www.ucalgary.ca/mrock). I especially thank Ann Toohey for providing critical feedback during the writing process, as well as Lydia Vaz for administrative assistance. I also thank the reviewers and the editors for this special issue of *Critical Public Health* on posthumanism.

Disclosure statement

No potential conflict of interest was reported by the author.

Funding

This work was supported by the Social Sciences and Humanities Research Council of Canada [grant number SRG-410-2004-2152]; the Alberta Heritage Foundation for Medical Research Endowment [grant number AHFMR-200600378]; and the Canadian Institutes of Health Research [grant number MSH-83745, grant number GIR-112745, grant number MOP-123380].

References

Agar, M. (2006). An ethnography by any other name …. *Forum: Qualitative Social Research, 7*. Retrived from http://www.qualitative-research.net/index.php/fqs/article/view/177

Bliss, M. (1982/2000). *The discovery of insulin* (2nd ed.). Toronto: University of Toronto Press.

Blue, G. (2015). Multi-species publics in the Anthropocene: From symbolic exchange to material-discursive intra-action. In Human Animal Research Network Editorial Collective (Ed.), *Animals in the anthropocene: Critical perspectives on non-human futures* (pp. 165–174). Sydney: Sydney University Press.

Blue, G., & Rock, M. J. (2011). Trans-biopolitics: Complexity in interspecies relations. *Health: An Interdisciplinary Journal for the Social Study of Health, Illness and Medicine, 15*, 353–368.

Blue, G., & Rock, M. (2014). Animal publics: Accounting for heterogeneity in political life. *Society & Animals, 22*, 503–519.

Christian, H., Bauman, A., Epping, J. N., Levine, G. N., McCormack, G., Rhodes, R. E., … Westgarth, C. (2016). A state of the art review: Encouraging dog walking for health promotion and disease prevention. *American Journal of Lifestyle Medicine*. doi:10.1177/1559827616643686.

City of Calgary. (2013). *Off-leash Area Management Plan, CPS2011-08. City of Calgary*, February 2011. Retrieved July 22, 2013, from http://www.calgary.ca/CSPS/Parks/Pages/Locations/Dog-off-leash-areas-in-parks.aspx#plan

City of Calgary. (2013). *Responsible Pet Ownership Bylaw: Protective Services Report to the Standing Policy Committee on Community and Protective Services*, CPS2006-08. City of Calgary, 21 February 2006. Retrieved July 22, 2013, from http://publicaccess.calgary.ca/lldm01/livelink.exe

Craddock, S., & Hinchliffe, S. (2015). One world, one health? Social science engagements with the one health agenda. *Social Science & Medicine, 129*, 1–4.

Cutt, H. E., Giles-Corti, B., Knuiman, M., & Burke, V. (2007). Dog ownership, health and physical activity: A critical review of the literature. *Health & Place, 13*, 261–272.

Degeling, C., & Rock, M. (2013). 'It was not just a walking experience': Reflections on the role of care in dog-walking. *Health Promotion International, 28*, 397–406.

Dewey, J. (1927/1991). *The Public and Its Problems*. Athens: Ohio University Press.

Durr, S., Mindekem, R., Kaninga, Y., Doumagoum Moto, D., Meltzer, M. I., Vounatsou, P., & Zinsstag, J. (2009). Effectiveness of dog rabies vaccination programmes: Comparison of owner-charged and free vaccination campaigns. *Epidemiology and Infection, 137*, 1558–1567.

Frohlich, K. L., & Abel, T. (2014). Environmental justice and health practices: Understanding how health inequities arise at the local level. *Sociology of Health & Illness, 36*, 199–212.

Frohlich, K. L., & Potvin, L. (1999). Health promotion through the lens of population health: Towards a salutogenic setting. *Critical Public Health, 9*, 211–222.

Fuentes, A. (2012). Ethnoprimatology and the anthropology of the human-primate interface. *Annual Review of Anthropology, 41*, 101–117.

Green, J. (2012). One health, one medicine, and critical public health. *Critical Public Health, 22*, 377–381.

Grier, K. C. (2006). *Pets in America: A history*. Chapel Hill: University of North Carolina Press.

Hansen, P. (2013). Urban Japan's "Fuzzy" new families: Affect and embodiment in dog–human relationships. *Asian Anthropology, 12*, 83–103.

Haraway, D. (2008). *When species meet*. Minneapolis, MN: University of Minnesota Press.

Headey, B., Na, F., & Zheng, R. (2007). Pet dogs benefit owners' health: A 'natural experiment' in China. *Social Indicators Research, 87*, 481–493.

Holmberg, T. (2013). Trans-species urban politics: Stories from a beach. *Space and Culture, 16*, 28–42.

Howell, P. (2012). Between the muzzle and the leash: Dog-walking, discipline, and the modern city. In P. Atkins (Ed.), *Animal cities: Beastly urban histories* (pp. 221–241). Burlington, VT: Ashgate Publishing Ltd.

Hurn, S. (2010). What's in a name? Anthrozoology, human-animal studies, animal studies or …? *Anthropology Today, 26*, 27–28.

Instone, L., & Sweeney, J. (2014). The trouble with dogs: 'Animaling' public space in the Australian city. *Continuum, 28*, 774–786.

Katz, J. (2006). Ethical escape routes for underground ethnographers. *American Ethnologist, 33*, 499–506.

Krieger, N. (2012). Who and what is a "population"? Historical debates, current controversies, and implications for understanding "population health" and rectifying health inequities. *Milbank Quarterly, 90*, 634–681.

Lail, P., McCormack, G., & Rock, M. (2011). Does dog-ownership influence seasonal patterns of neighbourhood-based walking among adults? A longitudinal study *BMC Public Health, 11*, 565. doi:https://bmcpublichealth.biomedcentral.com/articles/10.1186/1471-2458-11-148

Last, J. (Ed.). (2001). *A dictionary of epidemiology*. Oxford: Oxford University Press.

Maida, C. A., & Beck, S. (2015). Introduction. In S. Beck & C. A. Maida (Ed.), *Public anthropology in a borderless world* (pp. 1–35). New York, NY: Berghahn.

Marres, N. (2007). The issues deserve more credit: Pragmatist contributions to the study of public involvement in controversy. *Social Studies of Science, 37*, 759–780.

Marres, N. (2010). Front-staging nonhumans: Publicity as a constraint on the political activity of things. In B. Braun & S. J. Whatmore (Eds.), *Political matter: Technoscience, democracy and public life* (pp. 177–210). Minneapolis, MN: University of Minnesota Press.

Marres, N. (2016). The environmental teapot and other loaded household objects. In P. Harvey, E. Conlin Casella, G. Evans, H. Knox, C. McLean, E. B. Silva, N. Thoburn, & K. Woodward (Eds.), *Objects and materials: A Routledge companion* (pp. 260–272). Abington: Routledge.

Marres, N., & Lezaun, J. (2011). Materials and devices of the public: An introduction. *Economy and Society, 40*, 489–509.

Marsland, R. (2014). Who are the public in public health? Debating crowds, populations and publics in Tanzania. In R. J. Prince & R. Marsland (Eds.), *Making and unmaking public health in Africa: Ethnographic perspectives* (pp. 75–95). Athens: Ohio University Press.

Masuda, J. R., Poland, B., & Baxter, J. (2010). Reaching for environmental health justice: Canadian experiences for a comprehensive research, policy and advocacy agenda in health promotion. *Health Promotion International, 25*, 453–463.

Matisoff, D., & Noonan, D. (2012). Managing contested greenspace: Neighborhood commons and the rise of dog parks. *International Journal of the Commons, 6*, 28–51.

McCormack, G. R., Rock, M., Toohey, A. M., & Hignell, D. (2010). Characteristics of urban parks associated with park use and physical activity: A review of qualitative research. *Health & Place, 16*, 712–726.

McCormack, G. R., Shiell, A., Doyle-Baker, P. K., Friedenreich, C. M., & Sandalack, B. A. (2014). Subpopulation differences in the association between neighborhood urban form and neighborhood-based physical activity. *Health & Place, 28*, 109–115.

Nading, A.M. (2013). Humans, animals, and health: From ecology to entanglement. *Environment and Society: Advances in Research, 4*, 60–78.

Nading, A. M. (2014). *Mosquito trails: Ecology, health, and the politics of entanglement*. Berkeley: University of California Press.

Nutbeam, D. (1998). Health promotion glossary. *Health Promotion International, 13*, 349–364.

Parliament of Victoria. (2016). *Inquiry into the legislative and regulatory framework relating to restricted-breed dogs*, 2016/10/25/13:04:21. Retrieved October 25, 2016, from http://www.dogsvictoria.org.au/Portals/0/DOGS_Parliamentary%20Inquiry%20_report.pdf

Patrick, R., Dooris, M., & Poland, B. (2016). Healthy cities and the transition movement: Converging towards ecological well-being? *Global Health Promotion, 23*(Suppl 1), 90–93.

Pemberton, N., & Worboys, M. (2013). *Rabies in Britain: Dogs, disease and culture, 1830–2000*. London: Palgrave Macmillan.

Petersen, A. R. (1996). The 'healthy' city, expertise, and the regulation of space. *Health & Place, 2*, 157–165.

Richard, L., Gauvin, L., & Raine, K. (2011). Ecological models revisited: Their uses and evolution in health promotion over two decades. *Annual Review of Public Health, 32*, 307–326.

Rock, M. J. (2013). Pet bylaws and posthumanist health promotion: A case study of urban policy. *Critical Public Health, 23*, 201–212.

Rock, M., & Babinec, P. (2008). Diabetes in people, cats, and dogs: Biomedicine and manifold ontologies. *Medical Anthropology: Cross-Cultural Studies in Health and Illness, 27*(4), 324–352.

Rock, M., & Babinec, P. (2010). Prototypes connect human diabetes with feline and canine diabetes in the context of animal–human bonds: An anthropological analysis. *Anthrozoös: A Multidisciplinary Journal of the Interactions Between People and Animals, 23,* 5–20.

Rock, M. J. & Degeling, C. (2013). Public health ethics and a status for pets as person-things: Revisiting the place of animals in urbanized societies. *Journal of Bioethical Inquiry, 10,* 485–495.

Rock, M. J., & Degeling, C. (2015). Public health ethics and more-than-human solidarity. *Social Science & Medicine, 129,* 61–67.

Rock, M. J., & Degeling, C. (2016). Toward 'one health' promotion. In M. Singer (Ed.), *A companion to the anthropology of environmental health* (pp. 60–82). West Sussex: Wiley-Blackwell.

Rock, M. J., Adams, C. L., Degeling, C., Massolo, A., & McCormack, G. R. (2015). Policies on pets for healthy cities: A conceptual framework. *Health Promotion International, 30,* 976–986.

Rock, M. J., Degeling, C., Graham, T. M., Toohey, A. M., Rault, D., & McCormack, G. R. (2016a). Public engagement and community participation in governing urban parks: A case study in changing and implementing a policy addressing off-leash dogs. *Critical Public Health,* 1–14.

Rock, M. J., Graham, T. M., Massolo, A., & McCormack, G. R. (2016b). Dog-walking, dog-fouling and leashing policies in urban parks: Insights from a natural experiment designed as a longitudinal multiple-case study. *Landscape and Urban Planning, 153,* 40–50.

Rydin, Y., Bleahu, A., Davies, M., Dávila, J. D., Friel, S., De Grandis, G., … Wilson, J. (2012). Shaping cities for health: Complexity and the planning of urban environments in the 21st century. *The Lancet, 379,* 2079–2108.

Shibata, A., Oka, K., Inoue, S., Christian, H., Kitabatake, Y., & Shimomitsu, T. (2012). Physical activity of Japanese older adults who own and walk dogs. *American Journal of Preventive Medicine, 43,* 429–433.

Shortt, N. K., Rind, E., Pearce, J., & Mitchell, R. (2014). Integrating environmental justice and socioecological models of health to understand population-level physical activity. *Environment and Planning A, 46,* 1479–1495.

Smart, A. (2001). Restructuring in a North American city: Labour markets and political economy in Calgary. In M. W. Rees & J. Smart (Eds.), *Plural globalities in multiple localities: New world borders* (pp. 167–193). Lanham: University Press of America.

Smart, A. (2014). Critical perspectives on multispecies ethnography. *Critique of Anthropology, 34,* 3–7.

Smith, A. F., Semeniuk, C. A. D., Rock, M. J., & Massolo, A. (2015). Reported off-leash frequency and perception of risk for gastrointestinal parasitism are not associated in owners of urban park-attending dogs: A multifactorial investigation. *Preventive Veterinary Medicine, 120,* 336–348.

Srinivasan, K. (2013). The biopolitics of animal being and welfare: Dog control and care in the UK and India. *Transactions of the Institute of British Geographers, 38,* 106–119.

Tanasescu, A., Wing-tak, E. C., & Smart, A. (2010). Tops and bottoms: State tolerance of illegal housing in Hong Kong and Calgary. *Habitat International, 34,* 478–484.

Taylor, W. C., Floyd, M. F., Whitt-Glover, M. C., & Brooks, J. (2007). Environmental justice: A framework for collaboration between the public health and parks and recreation fields to study disparities in physical activity. *Journal of Physical Activity and Health, 4,* s50–s63.

Toohey, A. M., & Rock, M. J. (2011). Unleashing their potential: A critical realist scoping review of the influence of dogs on physical activity for dog-owners and non-owners. *International Journal of Behavioral Nutrition and Physical Activity, 8,* 46–54.

Toohey, A. M., & Rock, M. J. (2015). Newspaper portrayals, local policies, and dog-supportive public space: Who's wagging whom? *Anthrozoös, 28,* 549–567.

Toohey, A. M., McCormack, G. R., Doyle-Baker, P. K., Adams, C. L., & Rock, M. J. (2013). Dog-walking and sense of community in neighborhoods: Implications for promoting regular physical activity in adults 50 years and older. *Health & Place, 22,* 75–81.

Urbanik, J., & Morgan, M. (2013). A tale of tails: The place of dog parks in the urban imaginary. *Geoforum, 44,* 292–302.

Walsh, J. M. (2011). *Unleashed Fury: The political struggle for dog-friendly parks.* West Lafayette, IN: Purdue University Press.

Warner, M. (2002). Publics and counterpublics. *Public Culture, 14,* 49–90.

Westgarth, C., Gaskell, R. M., Pinchbeck, G. L., Bradshaw, J. W. S., Dawson, S., & Christley, R. M. (2009). Walking the dog: Exploration of the contact networks between dogs in a community. *Epidemiology and Infection, 137,* 1169–1178.

Westgarth, C., Christley, R. M., & Christian, H. E. (2014). How might we increase physical activity through dog walking?: A comprehensive review of dog walking correlates. *International Journal of Behavioral Nutrition and Physical Activity, 11,* 83–97.

World Health Organization (WHO). (1986). *Ottawa Charter for Health Promotion* [online]. Author. Retrived 20, 2012, from http://www.phac-aspc.gc.ca

Wolfe, C. (2010). *What is posthumanism?.* Minneapolis, MN: University of Minnesota Press.

Wood, L. J., Giles-Corti, B., & Bulsara, M. (2005). The pet connection: Pets as a conduit for social capital? *Social Science & Medicine, 61,* 1159–1173.

Wood, L. J., Giles-Corti, B., Bulsara, M. K., & Bosch, D. A. (2007). More than a furry companion: The ripple effect of companion animals on neighborhood interactions and sense of community. *Society & Animals, 15,* 43–56.

Zinsstag, J., Schelling, E., Waltner-Toews, D., & Tanner, M. (2011). From 'one medicine' to 'one health' and systemic approaches to health and well-being. *Preventive Veterinary Medicine, 101,* 148–156.

Enacting toxicity: epidemiology and the study of air pollution for public health

Emma Garnett

ABSTRACT

This paper presents air pollution as a 'post-human' public health phenomenon. It draws on an ethnography of a multidisciplinary research project called Weather Health and Air Pollution to explore the material ways in which air pollution challenged scientists' conceptualisations of harm and health. The epidemiologists on WHAP used statistical techniques to correlate data of air pollution concentrations with mortality and morbidity data collected by hospitals in order to establish a quantified measure of the health effects of exposure to air pollution. Initially, these correlations were problematic: plotted data points failed to map over temporal patterns. A series of negotiations followed. As a result of these, the concept of 'season' emerged as a temporal figure through which the very existence and meaning of air pollution was put to the test. Indeed, attempts by researchers to hold stable the notion of toxicity signalled the problem of trying to assess the bodily response to a polluted environment that has supposedly 'already been'. The paper concludes by arguing how contemplating health through the lens of the material dimensions of time allows public health to: first, view health problems as constituted through bodies and environments, rather than as a relation separating the two; and second, open up indeterminacies and uncertainties as a generative condition of air pollution, and perhaps public health more generally.

Introduction

[…] the environment is a world that continually *unfolds* in relation to the beings that make a living there … And as the environment unfolds, so the materials of which it is comprised do not *exist* – like the objects of the material world – but *occur* … They are neither objectively determined nor subjectively imagined but practically experienced. (Ingold, 2007, 14)

Air pollution is often framed as a complex social, political and environmental public health problem – an approach reflected in interdisciplinary funding opportunities, new policy committees, communities and proliferating academic and non-academic research collaborations. As a consequence, any sociological study of air pollution is inherently concerned with more-than-human relations. Air transgresses any distinction between 'humans' and 'the environment' because it is both external and internal to living, breathing bodies. Air pollution is, to use Haraway's term, a useful 'natureculture' (Haraway, 2003; Miele & Latimer, 2014; Whatmore, 2014): a proposition for re-writing modernist oppositions to illustrate the entanglement of the natural and the cultural, the body and the mind, the material and the semiotic.

This paper draws on ethnographic fieldwork of scientific research in action to explore what the nature–culture of air pollution opens up and forecloses in terms of understanding urban environments and human health relations. The setting was the Weather, Health and Air Pollution (WHAP)[1] project, a UK-based interdisciplinary scientific collaboration studying the epidemiological relationship between exposure to air pollutants and short-term health effects. Such initiatives, although recognising the interrelatedness of different factors, are often premised on the assumption that humans are separate from the natural environment, and that in order to respond to the problem of air pollution each first has to be studied independently. This plays out at different scales, from policy and governance initiatives that seek to change health behaviours or reduce fossil fuel emissions, to the everyday politics of scientific practice that collect data on either human health or atmospheric environments.[2]

Conceiving of air pollution as an inherently entangled kind of a phenomenon has wider consequences for public health science and practice because the contingencies that determine what counts as polluting and harmful, when, and how, means that it can only be understood through the inclusion of social *and* material, human *and* environmental processes and relations. But as Schrader (2010) points out, relational toxicities are not only contingent on social and material processes because they are also history-dependent. In other words, toxicity is tied up with time. This temporal aspect of pollution was a concern for WHAP researchers too, because their initial statistical patterns suggested air pollution is bad for you in winter but good for you in summer. This paradox arose because it was presumed toxicity must be directly locatable in the environment. Alternative scientific practices and modifications were therefore included in order to address the apparent discrepancy. Implicit in such a response was that some 'thing' in the environment is toxic because it contains an effect on human health within it (e.g. toxicity is independent of humans).

The focus of this paper will be on how exposure to air pollution is measured and enacted through scientific work in ways that demonstrate leaky boundaries (Nading, 2016) and the co-constitutive nature of human and non-human formations. Inspired by growing attention in Science and Technology Studies (STS) (Schrader, 2010; Murphy, 2013a, 2013b) and anthropology (Nading, 2016; Shapiro, 2015) to 'toxic relations', I will trace how measurements of health effects (toxic effects of exposure to air pollution) came about through scientists making particular connections and enacting particular exclusions (Schrader, 2010). This dynamic of inclusion and exclusion is an opportunity to explore how particular scientific practices, or the assembling of certain kinds of environment–health relations, enact toxicity in ways that do not always contain a dyadic relationship between cause and effect, environment and body. As the opening quotation from Ingold describes, the properties of materials are not fixed attributes but processual and relational. Process signifies the passage of time, flux and flow, which implicate human health in multiple and indeterminate ways.

I will begin by introducing the different data used by WHAP researchers and how the bringing together of these data generated problematic correlations. From there I will delve into the ethnographic detail of my argument, specifying the tensions and opportunities that the problem of air pollution posed in terms of generating statistically informed narratives and visually productive patterns of air pollution and health relationships. The final section will then consider the performative nature of statistical data practices, and how including more-than-human processes and temporalities can shift notions of pollution and toxicity, and environmental harm and health more generally.

Epidemiology of air pollution

Tim and Rob, two senior epidemiologists, were checking that a document being shared with the team displayed the correct results. These plotted data visualised an unexpected finding: air pollution is good for you in the summer and bad for you in the winter. Since the graphs illustrated these unlikely patterns further investigation was proposed, and a series of statistical manipulations and additional graphs were then discussed. (Fieldnotes, 20 January 2014)

A correlation is an association between two variables. A negative correlation means that as one variable (e.g. air pollution) increases the other variable (e.g. health effects) decreases. The assumption behind a times-series study[3] of air pollution is that each variable is a discrete bounded whole which interact inter-dependently, and that by relating the two patterns and associations can be captured and explained. The initial 'unlikely patterns' meant statistical methods had to be modified to ensure they were visualising the 'right relations' and thereby the relevant health risks associated with poor air quality.

Working out which relations are included or excluded in the construction and enactment of bodies and disease are central to many sociological studies of health and illness. The mundane work of assembling bodies and diseases is a particularly popular topic in STS inflected socio-material accounts of medicine and healthcare (Franklin, 2009; Martin, 2004; Mol, 2002; Mol & Law, 2004). These studies demonstrate the ways in which versions of health, disease and bodies are materialised and performed through practice. Numerical practices, like those of epidemiologists, are also performative (Hacking, 1990; Porter, 1996), because the defining of normative thresholds 'make up' (Hacking, 2007), classify (Bowker & Star, 1999) and privilege some bodies over others. Although the individual body is not always the locus of statistical work, assembling environmental and health data to understand risky and unhealthy air meant the boundaries and limits of bodies in relation to environments were explicitly played with and re-imagined by WHAP researchers.

Measuring the health effects of air pollution is intricately tied up with environmental governance and a rapidly growing network of monitoring and sensing devices across Europe and globally (Barry, 1998; Gabrys, 2016). With the increasing amounts of environmental data available, growing numbers of epidemiological studies are readily available for multiple air pollutants, with times-series studies in particular showing statistically significant associations between population-level exposure to air pollution and adverse health effects (Bingheng & Haidong, 2008, p. 5). Rather than focus on bodies or environments, I will examine how researchers on WHAP brought these phenomena together through statistical data practices. Large data-sets in combination with different methods, tools and analyses can foster new ways of seeing (Coopmans, Vertesi, Lynch, & Woolgar, 2014) whilst enacting phenomena in ways that enable novel investigation (Levin, 2014; Gitelman, 2013). Thus, after briefly introducing air pollution data and health data, I will discuss the ways in which the combining of data in scientific practices shifted human–environment relationships, whilst putting into question health as a relation which separates environments from bodies. This destabilisation and de-centring of the human in human health opens up new kinds of questions about environmental harm and encourages a more inclusive and materially informed understanding of public health.

Air samples

Air pollution monitors capture discrete, single-point measurements of different pollutants in time and space. Automatic fixed-cabin monitors draw air into their specialist equipment to separate the pollutant to be measured from other parts of air in the sample. There are around two hundred monitoring stations across the UK-generating data on key pollutants considered harmful for health, including particulate matter (PM), ozone (O_3), oxides of nitrogen (NOx), carbon monoxide (CO) and sulphur dioxide (SO_4). Measurements are made continuously; these are then calibrated and undergo a series of quality assurance tests before becoming publicly available data and information of air pollution. In WHAP, these data-sets were accessed through colleagues based at a nearby university.

Because air changes state and constitution temporally, from season to season, day to day, hour to hour, monitoring devices are set to take air samples continuously. This 'real-time' is an achievement that contains air in ways that makes it measurable within a bounded interval. It also constrains air pollution in paradoxical ways, because a moment of capture is a pause that cannot be experienced (Schrader, 2010 cf. Helmreich & Weston, 2006), which results in the construction of an absence between past and future moments (Schrader, 2010, p. 300). The 'lag' or latency (Murphy, 2013a) of chemical processes is also taken into account by monitoring site attendants and data analysers through quality assurance practices. Nonetheless, the relationship between air pollution in the atmosphere and a human breather being exposed to this same air is neither certain nor directly measurable. This discrepancy remained problematic for the epidemiologists because they were using monitored data as proxies for human exposure.

Health data

There were three types of health data-sets used on the project: national post-coded mortality data (2000–2010), post-coded Hospital Episode Statistics (2000/2001–2009/2010); and Myocardial Infarction National Audit Project (MINAP) data (2003–2009). The Office for National Statistics (ONS) collects information on cause of death from death certificates verified by civil registration records. The death registration also records a list of other conditions or diseases that the patient had at the time of death and which may be linked with the death, such as air pollution. The Hospital Episode Statistics is a data warehouse for records of all admissions, outpatient appointments and A&E attendances at NHS hospitals across England. This data is collected during a patient's time at hospital and provides information on illness, disease and outcome. MINAP is a clinical audit of hospital management of heart disease which provide specific disease mortality and outcome data.

Together, these cardiovascular-related morbidity and mortality data were linked with air pollution data in order to examine short-term health effects of exposure to air pollution (monitored data were the exposure data in this study). Short-term effects included mortality and morbidity counts resulting from exposure to air pollution on the same day and the days following a high air pollution episode. Linking back to the inevitable gap between the 'capture of air' and a 'real-time measurement' in monitoring, there is a dissonance here between exposure to air pollution and bodily affect. The temporal aspects of exposure to air pollution remained a challenge for researchers because of their need to separate particular kinds of bodies from particular kinds of air. For example, long-term risks like birth defects, cancer, degenerative disease and even poor mental health (Power et al., 2015), along with less measurable concerns, like wheezing and irritated eyes, were not included in this project. What kinds of bodily affects are measurable and considered of relevance shapes what counts as a health effect and thereby what constitutes toxic air. Body and environment relations are therefore pre-determined through the selection of environmental and health data.

Measuring exposure

Exposure was assumed to be the same as a measure of air pollution, and hospital data a way to measure the outcomes of exposure to air pollution concentrations on the same day. In time-series studies, repeated observations of air pollution and health (daily mortality or morbidity counts) are made, and analysis centres on comparing variations in these exposure–response patterns over the same time period (Bingheng & Haidong, 2008). Exposure is difficult to measure because data are only collected at specific points in space and time, yet personal exposure changes as individuals move around throughout the day. In addition, human bodies have different levels of sensitivity, and subsequent quantifications of health risk from exposure are steeped with uncertainty (Stilianakis, 2015). Although negotiations on WHAP involved accounting for the multiple disturbances that interrupted the epidemiologists' ability to measure exposure, the very implementation and use of environmental *and* human health data-sets pre-empted the empirical parameters for what could count as exposure in the first place. That these data-informed parameters became problematic for researchers meant notions of exposure and the stability of measures of health also required further examination. In the following sections, I map out the ways in which the problematic bringing together of environment and health data made the limits of perception tangible. Developing ways to perceive and materialise air pollution and health relations differently also fostered attempts to manage and contain air pollution and exposed bodies in more inclusive ways (thereby understanding body–air relations in 'other' ways).

Plotting correlations

On a scatter plot, a negative correlation displays data points clustered around a line from the top left-handside of the graph, and decreasing towards the bottom right-hand side corner of the graph.

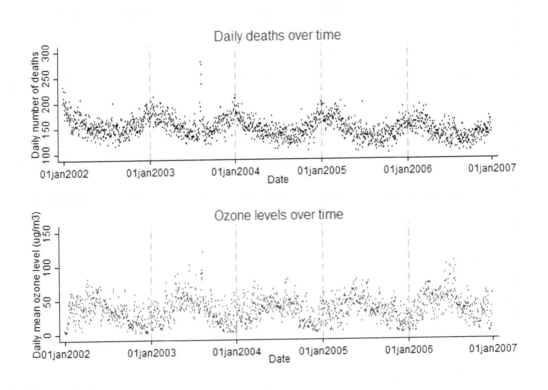

Figure 1. Illustrative STATA run: Two scatter plot which show the correlation between levels of ozone and mortality. Source: (Data from Bhaskaran et al. (2013).

The epidemiologists looked for correlations between the fluctuation of health events and air pollution episodes; of how many people died or how many hospital admissions occurred on a certain day in a bounded area. Mapping these correlations on scatter plots, they found the initial scatter plots problematic because they showed unexpected correlations. In summer air pollution levels and health effects appeared to be highly correlated, yet in winter they were less so, indicating that the same levels of air pollution may have different health effects at different times of the year. What was expected was an inverse relationship in both winter and summer, indicating that high levels of some pollutants are bad for health across seasons. The epidemiologists decided to test out their statistical methods to 'see what is really going on'. As one epidemiologist explained: 'the epi team are scratching their heads on this, about what we do in terms of these sharp distinctions between seasons?' (Peter, Meeting 20 January 2014).

The patterns on the graphs were a starting point for working out how to make perceptible the anticipated 'right relations' of air pollution and health. The problem was articulated through the plotted patterns and 'the wave' became a form itself, described as 'smooth', 'peaked', or 'dipped'. Implicit in these discussions was the assumption that it was the statistical work on data (of the variables of interest) that made the patterns appear like they did, rather than anything intrinsic about air pollution as a phenomenon. The patterns were not considered indicative of real causal relations, and it was hoped that through re-arranging the plotted data points clearer and simpler trends would be revealed. Specifically, the epidemiologists wanted to work out how 'season', recognised as a quality of the physical environment as well as a culturally constructed classification, was unduly influencing the scatter plots. In this way, season was considered a unit of time as well as a descriptor for the geo-physical annual cycle.

Tim, an epidemiologist, and Chris, an environmental chemist, discussed how to manage the passage of time and whether a conceptual re-framing of season in the epidemiologists' statistical model could solve the problematic correlations:

> Tim: yeah but my point is, on this, even though they are the traditional definitions of seasons they are still some-what arbitrary definitions of what a season is. And what I'm trying to work out, therefore, so what is the difference between autumn and winter?

> Chris: you are right they are a blunt distinction, I mean I guess it is convention, [but] you have to work with something (Meeting 20 January 2014).

Here, Tim proposes transgressing what he called 'traditional seasonal classifications' because autumn and winter are the same in terms of their interpretation of the initial scatter plots. Four seasons were thought to be interfering with the correlations, which is why Tim asks other team members: 'What is the difference between autumn and winter? Could health effects also be captured with a binary distinction of 'a warm summer and a cool winter'? By simplifying atmospheric changes over an annual year into temperature/two seasons, Tim and the other epidemiologists sought a simple way of finding and clarifying causality through the scatter plots.

'We can think through the patterns', Tim proposed. Using the case of $PM_{2.5}$ as a pollutant related to NO_2, (nitrogen dioxide) he asked what Chris had expected to see: 'all positive with different magnitudes, or some positive and negative, what would you have guessed?' Yet in response, a more attentive question towards the materiality of air and its entanglement with human health was presented:

> I would say [there is] higher $PM_{2.5}$ in summer, because you have contribution from secondary sources, in winter too, because you have a greater trapping of primary local sources. The composition will be different but the concentrations may be the same, but what impact this has on health, depends on what the causal exposure is between $PM_{2.5}$ and health. (Chris, Meeting 20 January 2014)

Although the epidemiologists considered splitting the passage of time to re-arrange statistical relationships in productive ways, this could not be done without taking responsibility for the material processes of atmospheric time and space. Indeed, from an environmental chemist's perspective, toxicity is not just a measure of a pollutant in the air, but results from a heterogeneous set of relations, including pollutant sources and wider atmospheric processes. These relations compose and re-compose air, which means the toxicity of air is an emergent attribute rather than stable thing.

From season as classification to season as materiality

The environmental chemists' interpretation of the irruption of season in the data patterns was that they signalled the larger mediating role of the atmosphere. This understanding complicated the initial interpretation of the results by the epidemiologists as being about the classification of the passage of time. Taking seriously the materiality of temporal processes meant, in many ways, the 'wrong' relations became 'right' because they were inclusive of the wider atmospheric processes shaping air pollution concentrations. As environmental chemist Chris had claimed, atmospheric processes and temporalities are tied up with 'short-term health effects' in ways that needed to be accounted for if exposure is to be accurately measured. Chris further challenged Tim and the epidemiologists' management of season, arguing that what season 'is' is not something you can just re-classify, because its materiality is entwined with emissions production and climatology. For example, primary sources in winter include emissions from fuel burning. In contrast, during summer months there are more secondary sources resulting from chemical reactions due to high temperatures and increased sunlight. It was not simply a re-configuring of the passage of time through season, but a shift in the epidemiologists' temporal framing of air pollution that was required.

It is difficult to include the passage of time and the emergence of air pollution in time-series analysis in any simple linear way, however. For example, seasonal patterns are particular to specific air pollutants, which influence the chemical properties of air and therefore levels of toxicity. Complicating the epidemiologists' argument that ozone is dependent on temperature in summer and winter seasons (and therefore that a binary seasonal distinction functions just as well as the traditional four season classification), Chris draws on the case of nitrogen dioxide, the chemical properties of which are tied-up with ozone.[4] He argues that exposure data should be understood in the context of the materiality of atmospheric processes, rather than relating directly and linearly to temperature:

> If we are not to throw in another complexity here, we're not told anything about NO_2, as well […] and that will have its own complex, annual cycles and variable interactions, or correlations, I'm sure, with ozone and particulate matter components. (Chris, Meeting 20 January 2014)

In this explanation, a more materially informed air pollution–health relationship is offered through the inclusion of atmospheric temporalities (tied up with but not solely defined by annual fluctuations and changes). Furthermore, relationships are not always proportional, and as temperature increases in summer air pollutants do not increase at the same rate. This suggests that pollutants also have their own temporalities, which makes the simplification of season as a unit of time and as a way to manage and understand air pollution–health relationships somewhat lacking.

The project's focus on short-term, acute health effects was challenged by the visibility of other atmospheric temporalities, yet by excluding long-term processes the materiality of short-term exposure also shifted. This disruption made other temporalities perceptible. As Murphy writes (2013a), it is through the distributed ways in which the chemicals of the past arrive in the present that taken for granted temporalities can be disrupted. The initial inclusion of long-term processes was therefore productive, because it highlighted how inclusions, and possible exclusions, shape correlations of interest. Accounting for the temporal dimension of air pollution meant that understandings of what becomes polluting in the air moved beyond an essentialist approach to the property of objects in the environments, to the ways in which toxicity of things move in and out of atmospheric 'time-space presents'. Exposure, then, was not simply a bodily response but on-going entanglements. Correlating air pollution and health data as discrete phenomena misses the ways in which toxicity occurs (Ingold, 2007) through these environment–body relations. Paying attention to the material contexts of air pollution and health, and significantly to their material histories and temporalities, opened up possibilities for exploring the varied pathways of chemical things as they permeate and structure life (Murphy, 2013a).

Statistical modifications

The shape of waves on a scatter plot affects their meaning: too few will fail to capture the general patterns, yet too many produces a weak visual pattern, reducing the power of future statistical claims by widening confidence intervals of relative risk estimates (Bhaskaran, Gasparrini, Hajat, Smeeth, & Armstrong, 2013, p. 1191). Scatter plots can display as 'wobbly waves', with too many variations to easily see the overall patterns, in comparison to 'smooth waves', which are more immediately comprehensible.

In this project, modifications to manage time more flexibly in time-series analyses were proposed in order to make short-term health effects more visible. The epidemiologists wanted to produce a 'smooth wave', and decided on fitting a cubic spline function to the original time-series model of a full seasonal year. Long-term patterns of four seasons had previously been modelled as a regular wave with single, equally spaced peaks and troughs. The cubic spline function was a way to manipulate the peaks and troughs in ways that reduced the dominance of material processes tied up with the cycle of a seasonal year.

A spline function consists of a number of sub-functions defined by 'polynomial variables' (variables which are indeterminate, like pollutant levels or temperature). By adding sub-functions to the initial time-series model, researchers could link together different 'pieces' or segments of time in ways that made time a more flexible variable, and with different capacities and affordances. The 'piecewise' process of cubic spline meant that a property of time (like temperature) holds for one part or piece of the time variable (linking these points smoothly) but not necessarily for the whole domain function, thereby dictating where a peak and trough may be situated. If time is stratified by month then the number of outcomes, that is the number of deaths or hospital admissions, will not be linked but independent in time. Without adding a cubic spline function, the graph jumps between increases or decreases in outcomes, with 'wobbly' features. These distract from the correlations the epidemiologists felt were evident between health outcomes and air pollution episode (across seasons, for example). A spline allows for the general trends of increases and decreases in mortality and morbidity counts to be understood in relation to one another rather than as discrete episodes. This results in the data points becoming less static, so that rather than a series of a-temporal correlations more complex and situated air pollution and health patterns can be detailed and explored.

Using the spline function allows peaks and troughs to be managed in ways that enable the perceived relevant patterns and associations to be visualised. For example, the initial estimate of a positive association between ozone levels and mortality risk was addressed by ensuring annual temperature did not dominate associations by scattering the points on a graph in ways that made patterns difficult to determine. By including the variable of temperature in the statistical model the differences between long and short term patterns could be better managed, and therefore short-term air pollution–health patterns further investigated and described. Modelling and controlling for the passage of time in this way reduced the dominance of long-term seasonal trends and moved the estimated ozone and mortality association towards the null, so that they were no longer statistically significant: they appeared as in the scatter plot in Figure 2. By making these patterns less visible 'the environment' became a smooth, stable background upon which health effects could be plotted and understood. A 'short-term' atmospheric environment was therefore constructed so that short-term health effects could be examined, but one that was inclusive of relations that made the correlations sensible and meaningful for both the epidemiologists and environmental chemists.

The statistical labour of managing these temporal interferences indicate once again the difficulty of separating bodies from environments in order to measure health. Significantly, what air pollution 'is', in terms of its relations to human harm and health, changed because exposure became the result of a set of atmospheric relations rather than a direct measure of an air pollutant (previously a proxy for exposure). Framing seasons in terms of warmer and cooler temperatures did not classify time in ways that revealed air pollution–health patterns correctly, because the practice of engaging with the correlations

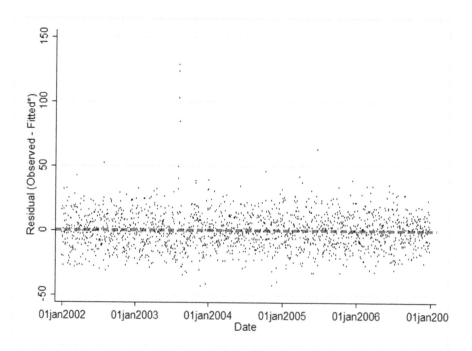

Figure 2. Illustrative STATA run: An adjusted visualisation with no peaks and no troughs. Source: Data from Bhaskaran et al. (2013).

demanded a reconfiguring of the meaning of toxicity. The initial attempt to make sense of the scatter plots by further simplifying time – from four seasons to two – was unsuccessful because it ignored the materiality of air pollution and atmospheric processes which characterise the passage of time.

There are other material processes entwined with temperature which further entangle material and human processes. $PM_{2.5}$, for example, is different in different seasons because in summer it is generated by secondary chemical reactions with gases like NO_2, and in winter it is a primary source generated by fuel burning to heat homes. Peter, an epidemiologist working alongside Tim, drew attention to the changing composition of this key pollutant of concern: 'if $PM_{2.5}$ is a different mixture in different seasons, could you argue the same for elemental carbon? We have elemental carbon here and isn't elemental carbon elemental carbon, whatever season?' (Meeting 20 January 2014). The case of carbon, as an element making up the heterogeneous pollutant $PM_{2.5}$, is used here to consider the patterns of difference within a pollutant specie, and thereby the differential effect of annual fluctuations and changes on air's composition and toxicity. A more particular and nuanced description of toxicity emerged, one that attended to the materiality of air in the generation of toxicity rather than the material attribute of the particle being inherently toxic.

Temporality and toxicity

I have described how epidemiologists constructed health patterns through statistical techniques and data plots (Figures 1 and 2). These outputs were not only representational, but used to actively interrogate and re-configure air pollution's form and meaning (Levin, 2013; Myers, 2008). Initially, statistical practices assumed the environment to be a stable background upon which outcomes of exposure could be marked and measured. But when work began to trace changes over time, the idea of exposure as referring to a bounded human body in a pre-existing atmospheric environment came undone. The result was that measuring the health effects of air pollution demanded the inclusion of changing atmospheres, chemical properties and geo-solar processes in ways that unfolded 'non-human' processes into 'human' ones (Nading, 2016).

Key in this development was an eventual recognition of the temporal instability of the toxicity of air and what it means in terms of harm and human health. Although the epidemiologists remained interested in the short-term effects of exposure, this negated the existence of other kinds of temporalities upon which the very moment of 'short-term' was contingent. This demanded the inclusion of season as a key concept, not in terms of 'cultural time' (the classifications we impose on the world) or 'natural time' (material fluctuations in the world), but as 'material-cultural time' (human behaviour and geo-solar cycles). Through the inclusion of socio-material processes of season and emissions, the chemistry and epidemiology of atmospheric air were related to health data in ways that demonstrated the contingency of pollution. For example, by suggesting it was possible to understand the seasonal effects of particulate matter on health through a stable particle like black carbon, the epidemiologists began to use time to read air pollution[5]. Indeed, accounting for temporalities which were in excess of human time and certain kinds of bodily effects extended relations of health to include the chemical species and geo-solar processes which compose human bodies and shape patterns of exposure.

By responding to non-human agencies through statistical work and visual plots, the formulation of different kinds of questions about environmental harm and human health were made possible. The more-than-human matter of time, as a thicker kind of materiality (Puig de la Bellacasa, 2011), enabled a broader framing of exposure. The changes in the graph were a response to other rhythms, qualities and forces (Stewart, 2011), leading to a shift in the temporal ordering of environment–bodies through the modification of statistical tools and techniques. First, this meant that the toxic, or not, qualities of the chemical constituents of air became spatially contingent but also temporally dependent (Schrader, 2010). And second, by pursuing the temporal qualities of air the notion of bodily exposure shifted to include ongoing human–material processes and encounters – from the deep geo-solar shifts that influence daylight hours and temperature, to the ways in which emissions ebb and flow as a result of human behaviour. Questioning the arrangement of seasonal time meant taking seriously the mediating role of atmospheric processes and the entanglement of environment–human relations. Rather than something that could be ignored, the variable of time therefore became essential to understanding air pollution and health correlations. Accordingly, exposure became situated in time, and season a unit of time through which air pollution could also be investigated.

Concluding discussion

Incorporating material processes which define the passage of time into measures of everyday human health complicated any stable relationship between bodies and environments. Reminiscent of Ingold's anecdote about air and fog, researchers had to shift between technical practice and material enactment: 'When the fog descends, and everything around you looks dim and mysterious, has the material world changed, or are you just seeing the same world differently?' (Ingold, 2011, p. 21). By re-considering season as a unit of time in epidemiological data practices the material qualities of air changed. At the same time, the environmental chemists were keen to ensure the team weren't just seeing the same world through the fog of ill-plotted graphs and inadequate statistical functions. The tensions involved in working through statistical correlations that demonstrate the fluctuating indeterminate world, whilst developing statistical techniques inclusive of these material processes, was managed through the introduction of a cubic spline function.

Social and cultural theorists of air have described how defining elements in terms of their epistemological or ontological definition, and thereby distinction and separation, may miss their inherent qualities as 'mediation' (Adey, 2015; Connor, 2010) and as 'a gathering force' (Ingold, 2012; Martin, 2011). But as Nading argues, the entanglement between human and nonhuman need not be a problem for public health to overcome but a starting point for understanding health itself (2016, p. 4). Although controlling for season silenced long-term patterns, ultimately making them less visible in the plotted data points, its labour and practice actively engaged with the materiality of air and the changing composition of the atmosphere over time. In this way, statistical practices of visualisation and modification enabled researchers to engage with and conceptualise air pollution as entangled entities. Indeed, it wasn't just the work of making and making sense of data that the problem of season encouraged, but the dialogue it generated between the environmental chemists and epidemiologists that was co-productive of data analysis and interpretation. Rather than the visual work of scientists distancing and objectifying 'health' through measures of risk, I have drawn attention to the thickening entanglements of scientists as they sought an adequate statistical model for capturing and explaining air pollution–health relations beyond cause and effect, environment and body.

Air pollution is an unruly public health problem, yet its hybridity and ongoing entanglement can instigate new ways of thinking about the relations beween environmental harm and health (Will, 2017). Instead of simple graphs I have shown how a range of statistical and visual practices enacted toxicity in ways that re-arranged these relationships, affording new epistemic capacities and understandings. Focusing on the intrarelatedness of bodies and environments through data practices was a way to explore the re-making of socio-material and temporal scales, and the ways in which it redressed the underlying assumptions initially framing air pollution in WHAP. The practice of thinking from within the material world, and not from a position outside, can lead to the inclusion of human and non-human encounters: from the perspective of chemical reactions to the more standard mortality and morbidity statistics. In this way, by comprehending air pollution through the contingency of social *and* material processes the environment is no longer merely a context from which human health can be improved, but an active space for its re-imagination and re-configuration.

Notes

1. All names are psuedonyms.
2. The WHAP project was considered novel by team members in its bringing together and linking of environmental data with health data.

3. Time-series data are data collected on the same observational unit at multiple time periods. In time-series regression analysis, variations in exposure status are compared with changes in health outcomes in a given area.
4. Nitrogen dioxide (NO_2) is a key pollutant of concern because of its inflammatory effects on the respiratory system. Both NO_2 and O_3 are intimately linked through atmospheric chemistry and continuously interchange over very short timescales (Williams, Atkinson, Anderson, & Kelly, 2014).
5. Thank you to one of the anonymous reviewers for this insight.

Acknowledgements

Special thanks to researchers on the WHAP project whose patience and support made this research possible. Thanks also to Judy Green and Simon Cohn for guidance during the PhD on which this work is based, and to Rebecca Lynch, Simon Cohn and the two anonymous reviewers for their thoughtful and productive comments on earlier versions of this paper. Ethical approval was granted by the London School of Hygiene & Tropical Medicine Ethics Committee.

Disclosure statement

No potential conflict of interest was reported by the author.

Funding

The author received doctoral funding from The Natural Environment Research Council, UK [grant number NE/I007938/1]. Financial support was also received from the Foundation for the Sociology of Health and Illness, which assisted the writing of this paper.

References

Adey, P. (2015). Air's affinities: Geo-politics, chemical affect, and the force of the elemental. *Dialogues in Human Geography, 5*, 54–75.
Barry, A. (1998). *Motor ecology: The political chemistry of urban air*. London: Goldsmiths College.
Bhaskaran, K., Gasparrini, A., Hajat, S., Smeeth, L., & Armstrong, B. (2013). Time series regression studies in environmental epidemiology. *International Journal of Epidemiology, 42*, 1187–1195.
Bingheng, C., & Haidong, K. (2008). Air pollution and population health: A global challenge. *Environmental Health and Preventive Medicine, 13*, 94–101.
Bowker, G. C., & Star, S. L. (1999). *Sorting things out: Classification and its consequences*. Cambridge, MA: MIT Press.
Connor, S. (2010). *The matter of air: Science and art of the ethereal*. London: Reaktion.
Coopmans, C., Vertesi, J., Lynch, M., & Woolgar, S. (2014). Introduction: Representation in scientific practice revisited. In C. Coopmans, J. Vertesi, M. Lynch, & S. Woolgar (Eds.), *Representation in scientific practice revisited* (pp. 1–12). Cambridge, MA: MIT Press.
Franklin, S. (2009). Genetic bodies. In A. Herle, M. Elliot, & R. Empson (Eds.), *Assembling bodies: Art, science and imagination* (pp. 66–67). Cambridge: Cambridge Museum of Archaeology and Anthropology.
Gabrys, J. (2016). *Program earth: Environmental sensing technology and the making of a computational planet*.
Gitelman, L. (Ed.). (2013). *"Raw data" is an oxymoron*. London: MIT University Press.
Hacking, I. (1990). *The taming of chance*. Cambridge: Cambridge University Press.
Hacking, I. (2007). Kinds of people: Moving targets. *Proceedings of the British Academy, 151*, 285–318.
Haraway, D. (2003). *The companion species manifesto: Dogs, people, and significant otherness*. Chicago, IL: Prickly Paradigm Press.
Helmreich, S., & Weston, K. (2006). Gender in real time: Power and transience in a visual age. *Body and Society, 12*, 103–121.
Ingold, T. (2007). Materials against materiality. *Archaeological Dialogues, 14*, 1–16.
Ingold, T. (2011). *Being alive: Essays on movement, knowledge and description*. Abingdon: Routledge.
Ingold, T. (2012). Towards an ecology of materials. *Annual Review of Anthropology, 41*, 427–442.
Levin, N. (2013). *Enacting molecular complexity: Data and health in the metabonomics laboratory* (PhD). Oxford: Social Anthropology, Oxford University.
Levin, N. (2014). Multivariate statistics and the enactment of biological complexity in metabolic science. *Social Studies of Science, 44*, 555–578.
Martin, E. (2004). *Flexible bodies: Tracking immunity in american culture from the days of polio to the age of AIDS*. Boston, MA: Beacon Press Books.
Martin, C. (2011). Fog-bound: Aerial space and the elemental entanglements of body-with-world. *Environment & Planning D: Society & Space, 29*, 454–468.

Miele, M., & Latimer, J. (2014). Natureculture's? Science, affect and the non-human. *Theory Culture and Society, 30*, 5–31.

Mol, A. (2002). *The body multiple: Ontology in medical practice*. Durham: Duke University Press.

Mol, A., & Law, J. (2004). Embodied action, enacted bodies: The example of hypoglycaemia. *The Body and Society, 10*, 43–62.

Murphy, M. (2013a). Distributed reproduction, chemical violence, and latency. *Scholar and Feminist Online, 11*, 3.

Murphy, M. (2013b). Chemical infrastructures of the St. Clair River. In S. Boudia & N. Jas (Eds.), *Toxicants, health and regulation since 1945* (pp. 103–116). London: Pickering & Chatto Publishers.

Myers, N. (2008). Molecular embodiments and the body-work of modeling in protein crystallography. *Social Studies of Science, 38*, 163–199.

Nading, A. (2016). Local biologies, leaky things, and the chemical infrastructure of global health. *Medical Anthropology*, 1–16. Ahead of Print. doi:10.1080/01459740.2016.1186672

Porter, T. M. (1996). *Trust in numbers: The pursuit of objectivity in science and public life*. Princeton, NJ: Princeton University Press.

Power, M. C., Kioumourtzoglou, M.-A., Hart, J. E., Okereke, O. I., Laden, F., & Weisskopf, M. G. (2015). The relation between past exposure to fine particulate air pollution and prevalent anxiety: Observational cohort study. *BMJ, 350*, h1111.

Puig de la Bellacasa, M. (2011). Matters of care in tecnoscience: Assembling neglected things. *Social Studies of Science, 41*, 85–106.

Schrader, A. (2010). Responding to pfiesteria piscicida (the fish killer): Phantomatic ontologies, indeterminacy, and responsibility in toxic microbiology. *Social Studies of Science, 40*, 275–306.

Shapiro, N. (2015). Attuning to the chemosphere: Domestic formaldehyde, bodily reasoning, and the chemical sublime. *Cultural Anthropology, 30*, 368–393.

Stewart, K. (2011). Atmospheric attunements. *Environment and Planning D: Society and Space, 29*, 445–453.

Stilianakis, N. I. (2015). *Susceptibility and vulnerability to health effects of air pollution: The case of nitrogen dioxide*. Joint Research Centre European Commission.

Whatmore, S. (2014). Earthly powers and affective environments: An ontological politics of flood risk. *Theory, Culture and Society, 30*, 33–50.

Will, C. (2017). On difference and doubt as tools for critical engagement with public health. *Critical Public Health, 27*, 293–302.

Williams, M. L., Atkinson, R. W., Anderson, H. R., & Kelly, F. J. (2014). Associations between daily mortality in London and combined oxidant capacity, ozone and nitrogen dioxide. *Air Quality, Atmosphere & Health, 7*, 407–414.

The injecting 'event': harm reduction beyond the human

Fay Dennis

ABSTRACT

Since the 1980s, the primary public health response to injecting drug use in the UK has been one of harm reduction. That is, reducing the harms associated with drug use without necessarily reducing consumption itself. Rooted in a post-Enlightenment idea of rationalism, interventions are premised on the rational individual who, given the right means, will choose to avoid harm. This lies in stark contrast to dominant addiction models that pervade popular images of the 'out of control' drug user, or worse, 'junkie'. Whilst harm reduction has undoubtedly had vast successes, including challenging the otherwise pathologising and often stigmatising model of addiction, I argue that it has not gone far enough in addressing aspects of drug use that go beyond 'rational' and 'human' control. Drawing on my doctoral research with people who inject drugs, conducted in London, UK, this paper highlights the role of the injecting 'event', which far from being directed or controlled by a pre-defined individual or 'body' was composed by a fragile assemblage of bodies, human and nonhuman. Furthermore, in line with the 'event's' heterogeneous and precarious make-up, multiple ways of 'becoming' through these events were possible. I look here at these 'becomings' as both stabilising and destabilising ways of being in the world, and argue that we need to pay closer attention to these events and what people are actually in the process of becoming in order to enact more accountable and 'response-able' harm reduction.

Introduction

> We assert our attachment to the species as if it were a matter of fact, a given. So much so that we construct a fundamental notion of Rights around the Human. But is it so? (Braidotti, 2013, p. 1)

The privileged position of the Human is evident in Public Health, with its place in harm reduction being no exception. Indeed, much of harm reduction's authority is based on a human right to health (Jürgens, Csete, Amon, Baral, & Beyrer, 2010). Exploring harm reduction's past, present and potential future, this paper hopes to outline and disrupt a reliance on the human and where it may be limiting a more open approach to drug–body relations and their effects. Through participants' narratives of injecting drugs, I aim to explore where the human unravels and new forms of relations and subjectivities come into being. Drawing on two concepts in particular – 'the event' and 'becoming' – I will highlight the many bodies, human and nonhuman, involved in injecting events, and the more-than-human bodies enacted, to the point that disentangling these oscillating processes becomes almost impossible. Following this disruption, I will then use the concepts of 'contingency' and 'care' to rebuild optimism in a harm reduction that no longer requires a bounded human, and instead strives to attune to these human and nonhuman *processes*, to reconfigure bodies in 'healthier' ways.

Harm reduction: a 'rational' drug policy and its critique

At the *First International Conference on the Reduction of Drug Related Harm,* in Liverpool, UK, in 1990 (Erickson, Riley, Cheung, & O'Hare, 1997, p. 7), delegates called for drug policy with less moralism and more *rationalism* (O'Hare, Newcombe, Matthews, Buning, & Drucker, 1991). In keeping with the new Public Health movement of the time, harm reduction activists called for the approach to be rooted in evidence (Erickson et al., 1997, p. 7). Indeed, the title of the book that emerged from the third conference on drug-related harm was entitled 'Psychoactive Drugs and Harm Reduction: *From Faith to Science*' (Heather, Wodak, Nadelmann, & O'Hare, 1993, my emphasis).

Importantly for this paper, the rationalism of the approach has produced an anthropocentrism. It is widely felt that if people who use drugs are given the correct evidence-based information and equipment they will make rational decisions based on internal cost/benefit analyses to reduce the harms associated with their drug use (Rumbold, Kellehear, & Hamilton, 1998; for critiques, see Mugford, 1993; O'Malley & Valverde, 2004). As such, The Human Rights Act has been used increasingly to substantiate these aims (Ezard, 2001; Hathaway, 2001; Hunt, 2004; Kerr, Wood, Betteridge, Lines, & Jürgens, 2004; Stevens, 2011), including specific calls for needle exchange programmes, opiate substitution treatment and, more recently, supervised injecting clinics and drug consumption rooms (e.g. Malinowska-Sempruch & Gallagher, 2004; Release, 2016; UNAIDS, 2015). Summed up in a review of the evidence on human rights abuses and vulnerability to HIV infection in *The Lancet*, Jürgens et al. (2010) states that a rights-based response to drug use must be taken.

However, a focus on *human* rights as a productive recourse for harm reduction has not been accepted by all. Keane (2003) cautions us that 'human rights may not be politically efficacious in the arena of drug use' (p. 227). In fact, she argues, 'they may work to reinforce a universal model of the "normal" sovereign individual ["at the core of what it is to be human"] that pathologises and marginalises drug users' (2003, p. 228). Instead, drawing on Isabelle Stengers (with Olivier Ralet, 1997), Keane argues for an 'ethical perspective based on open-ended debate, practices of freedom and a respect for difference' (2003, p. 228). I will return to this important interjection towards the end of the paper, but, for now, it is important to note that Keane's critique can be seen located in a wider counter-narrative concerned with how harm reduction could be perpetuating an individualising neoliberal agenda. For example, even as early as the third *International Conference on the Reduction of Drug Related Harm,* Mugford (1993) questioned the 'naivety of "liberation"' and 'limits of "reason"' (p. 31). Taking up a Foucauldian governmentality perspective, Mugford and other commentators in the social sciences criticise harm reduction policies and technologies for their disciplining effects (Bergschmidt, 2004; Bourgois, 2000; McLean, 2011; Miller, 2001; O'Malley & Valverde, 2004). In response to this critique, a 'social science *for* harm reduction' seeks to account for the social, economic and political influences in people's lives and decision-making (Rhodes, 2009) using concepts such as 'situated rationality' and 'risk environment' (Rhodes, 2002; Rhodes, Singer, Bourgois, Friedman, & Strathdee, 2005).

More recently, researchers have worked to dismantle the individualising tendencies of harm reduction even in its strategic and situated capacity (Moore & Fraser, 2006). Indeed, influenced by actor–network theory (ANT), and science and technology studies (STS) more broadly, the field has been said to be experiencing a 'material turn' (Duff, 2013; Seear & Moore, 2014). Ontologically, flatter conceptualisations of drug taking have emerged that seek to displace the 'drug taker', traditionally at the heart of research and policy, with wider notions of agency and who/what acts. For example, notably, Suzanne Fraser and colleagues look at how drugs, bodies and services in different space–time produce new subjectivities (Fraser, 2006; Fraser & Valentine, 2008), substances (Fraser & Valentine, 2006), conditions and diseases (Fraser, 2004; Fraser & Seear, 2011) and call for responses to be receptive to these collaborations and differences (Dwyer, Fraser, & Treloar, 2011; Fraser, Rance, & Treloar, 2016; Fraser, Treloar, Bryant, & Rhodes, 2014).

Although some of these 'posthuman' interests are long-standing (e.g. Gomart & Hennion, 1999), they are still not widespread or uncontroversial. Thus, I hope to help substantiate these trends in offering case examples from my research on injecting drug use to show: first, where the individual becomes undone; second, how other more-than-human formations emerge; and third, what alternative forms of policy and practice are therefore required.

Theoretical approach

> We believe in a world in which individuations are impersonal, and singularities are pre-individual. (Deleuze, 2004, p. xix)

Gilles Deleuze's philosophy of transcendental empiricism underpins my approach to 'the event' and 'becoming' taken in this paper. For Deleuze, life does not start with forms or organisms but these differences are produced in the process of life. 'The event' speaks to these moments where individuations come into being. Where the rationalism of harm reduction is based on the anterior human, an events perspective is underpinned by a relational and processual ontology, with the human always caught in the ebbs and flows of becoming. Those researching within the sociology of drug use have utilised 'the event' predominantly through Bruno Latour (e.g. Demant, 2009; Dilkes-Frayne, 2014; Duff, 2012; Gomart & Hennion, 1999; Race, 2015), and less so, through Gabriel Tarde (Bøhling, 2014; Vargas, 2010), Alfred Whitehead (Race, 2014), and Deleuze (Duff, 2014; Malins, 2004).

In Mike Michael's reading of Mariam Fraser's (2011) analysis of the 'event' at the intersections of STS and Deleuzian philosophy, he suggests there are two versions of the event at play:

> In one version, the event is characterized by a 'being with', where the constituents of the event 'co-habit' in the process of that event, interacting with, but not changing in relation to, one another. Alternatively, the event is marked by a 'becoming-with', where constituents themselves mutually change, or intra-act as Barad (2007) phrases it. (2015, p. 88)

Where drug events have been traced according to ANT, attention is paid to 'mediation' (e.g. Demant, 2009; Dilkes-Frayne, 2014; Duff, 2012; Race, 2015), and the moments these relational activities occur. This is seen to shift attention from 'who acts' to 'what occurs' (Dilkes-Frayne, 2014; Duff, 2016; Gomart & Hennion, 1999). For me, thinking with Deleuze shifts this focus to 'what becomes'. So a new question arises in terms of 'what becomings' or 'becoming-with drugs' (Michael & Rosengarten, 2012) *move* through the event?

The hyphen in 'becoming-with drugs' is important as it highlights that there are no pre-defined bodies – 'the body' or 'drug' – but these come to 'matter' (in its dual sense) in relation to each other. As Deleuze points out, 'mixtures are in bodies, and in the depth of bodies':

> A body penetrates another and coexists with it in all of its parts, like a drop of wine in the ocean, or fire in iron. [...] But what we mean by 'to grow', 'to diminish', 'to become red', 'to become green', 'to cut', and 'to be cut' etc. [...]. These are no longer states of affairs – mixtures deep inside bodies – but incorporeal events at the surface which are the results of these mixtures. The tree 'greens'. (Deleuze, 1990, pp. 5–6)

Using the infinitive form, Deleuze is distinguishing the event – 'greening' – from the tree and greenness. Therefore, as Stagoll points out, 'the event is not a disruption of some continuous state, but rather the state is constituted by events "underlying" it that, when actualised, mark every moment of the state as a transformation' (2010, p. 90). 'Becoming' moves through events, produced by and producing a connectivity in which participants express a certain 'becoming-together' or (noted by Michael above) as Karen Barad (2007) says, 'intra-action'. Where an 'interaction' suggests an encounter between two predefined bodies, an 'intra-action' acknowledges the relationality of those bodies that are pre-individually relational, so that, crucially for this paper, living singularly is always a product of multiplicity.

Aims and methods

The overarching aims of the PhD project drawn upon in this paper were to explore experiences and embodiments of injecting drug use that surpass cognitive, rational decision-making, whilst also complicating a dominant scientific narrative of addiction that erases much of the associated complexities. These aims have specific relevance to the current paper because as I explored these 'a-rational' (neither non-rational nor rational but simply otherwise to rational) accounts further, 'the human' subject started to dissipate, moving beyond its boundaries that proved porous, into the 'outside' and back in again. Participants described a unique exposure to the world as both painful and pleasurable: a discomfort or awkwardness with the 'outside' in experiences of being 'on edge', feeling that environments were 'too close' and/or '[sensorially] overloaded', but also an unrivalled affinity with the 'outside' that made people feel 'at one', 'blissful' and even like they were 'floating on air' – a truly dissipated state where boundaries between the outside and inside become almost entirely removed.

Even though I employed mostly conventional 'representational' methods to address these aims, in the liveliness of the research, they took me in nonrepresentational directions, which de-centred the subject, dislodged meaning-making and elided subject/object dualisms. These methods included interviews with 30 people who inject drugs, interviews with 10 managers and workers in two drug services, and a six-month placement in one of the services carrying out participant observation. Here, I draw mostly from the former interviews. These lasted approximately 1.5 hours and participants were reimbursed £15 for their time and travel costs. All participants identified as current injectors (having injected within the past four weeks), with the vast majority regularly injecting heroin and/or crack cocaine. I spoke to both men (n20) and women (n10), who were aged between 24 and 60 years, and from a range of social and ethnic backgrounds. Ethical approval was granted by the London School of Hygiene & Tropical Medicine Ethics Committee (ref. 7039) and the National Health Service Regional Ethics Committee (ref. 14/LO/0184).

Through these methods, my attention was drawn away from the 'individual' and towards a relation-ality of bodies, including genetic, material (nonhuman), imaginary and even institutional bodies, and how these more-than-human bodies were enacted through these assemblages. As such, the primary unit of analysis shifted from the spoken word of the drug user to the drug-using event. These directions were particularly aided through the use of body mapping. Whilst body mapping has been used to describe a number of practices, from a trauma therapy tool (Crawford, 2010) to 3D computer imaging (Tarr & Thomas, 2011), it refers here to a creative drawing method.

Participants were asked to draw their bodies in relation to how they felt before, during and after injecting drugs, and the people and things around them at the time. It was soon clear that rather than merely reflecting injecting experiences, the mapping process was actively involved in producing these realities – reorganising temporal patterns and bodily arrangements. Where talking in interviews largely forces events into a linear narrative, drawing allowed for alterative forms. Time, for instance, became rearranged topologically as spaces like the 'crack house' slowed time down. One participant said: 'the "gouching" [relaxed intoxication] time depends on … if I'm with people in a crack house, I don't really know them and that, then I can't relax in there'. Such findings tie in with other explorations of drug con-texts in which time and space are seen as co-constitutive (e.g. Bøhling, 2014; Duff, 2007, 2012; Farrugia, 2015; Fraser, 2006; Race, 2014). The drawings also rearranged the classic body with new boundaries drawn up between the inside and outside, where substances, for example, could be part of the inside (see Dennis, 2016b). Participants commented on an epidermal breakdown when they were drug-free: 'I'm a complete nervous wreck. I'll be jumping everywhere'; 'I don't want to be in my own skin'. One participant expressed feelings of 'disembodiment', of not feeling in his own body. Consequently, in the mapping process, bodies got redrawn *with* substances as well as other materials. To use Lury and Wakeford's (2012) heuristic, the body maps provided a 'device' into these more-than-human worlds.

> Devices act as a hinge between concepts and practice, epistemology and ontology, the virtual and the actual, [and help us] to recognise that knowledge practices, technical artefacts and epistemic things are encoded in everyday and specialised technologies and assemblages in which agency is no longer the sole privilege of human actors. (Lury & Wakeford, 2012, p. 9)

Therefore, from my starting point with an interest in going beyond the 'rational', I was *moved* through the research process yet further away from these human processes to the point that the human started to make little sense. Far from controllable or rational, the injecting event was a fragile sociomaterial achievement, involving both human and nonhuman processes, where new more-than-human bodies were also made. The remainder of the paper will deal with these two key findings and how they disrupt and reorganise our approach to drugs that rely too heavily on a distinction between drugs, bodies and environments, and the rational/irrational *drug user* who 'successfully' or 'unsuccessfully' navigates this interaction.

'On the tilt': the injecting event as a fragile achievement

> I suppose it's like having the worst hunger or anything and, or, you haven't had a drink for days and then you get water, and it's almost as if it could *drop over* at any minute, so you're really thirsty, so *it's on the tilt*, but if you get it then you're replenished, but if you miss it then it's on the floor. So it's the same if you miss a hit. (Lucy)

Lucy's narrative and body map, which has also proved useful in highlighting the trigger assemblage that moved her towards using drugs (see Dennis, 2016a; body map republished with permission), is used here to describe the fragility of the injecting event itself. She uses the analogy of the tilting water glass to describe a situation in which the 'success' of injecting is beyond her control ('could drop over at any minute'). Whether the injecting event comes together to enact 'success' – 'then you're replenished' – or failure – 'it's on the floor' – is, she goes on to explain, dependent on the precise coming together of a vast array of things, which she attempts to explore in her drawing (Figure 1).

In the picture (Figure 1), Lucy writes the words 'long term use, success, wonderful', by which to sum up a long discussion on the fragility of the injecting event. She makes clear to me that its 'success' is made up of several tentative bodies, body parts, substances, things, thoughts and words. Here, I look at the role of her hands, 'boyfriend', citric, blood, syringe and the techno-corporeal skills involved in keeping these connections together.

Lucy draws two pairs of hands. She explains that her hands play a vital role in the injecting event as the only area where she is able/willing to find a vein. She also notes the role that her boyfriend plays in helping her to inject.

> Because I always had problems injecting myself, I found it easier for him to do it for me. It was weird. I could do everything, but from that perspective, I had more luck if he was doing it […] It's almost like a wasted skill. He really should be in the profession of nursing, or something.

'Blood' is also prominently written in the body map, and is said to be a key actor in the 'success' of the injecting event. That is, she explains, a flush of blood in the syringe lets Lucy *know* that the needle is in the vein so the syringe can be plunged and its load released. The itchiness of the citric acid is similarly noted in the picture, which she uses to dissolve the heroin into an injectable solution. Although it is uncomfortable, it is necessary for indicating that the mixture has gone into the vein, without which she would be unsure and not fully able to enjoy it.

> Citric gives an itchy sensation, but you *know* when you get this itchy, it's weird, it's actually uncomfortable, but you *know* that you've had a successful hit. Even if you go, 'oh itchy, I need to go and wash my hand', it's like intense pins and needles, you know that the citric has gone in, it's gone in, it's worked, so you know that soon after you're starting to do that (nod off). Even though you're annoyed, it's a horrible itchy feeling, because it's the citric going into your veins. With Vitamin C, it's less itchy, but what I've noticed with the itchy feeling is the success. It always

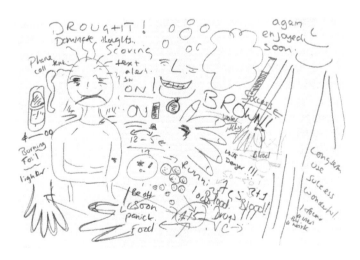

Figure 1. Lucy's body map.

means it's pulled well, it hasn't hurt and it's worked, so success. So 'itchy, success', and then I'd go to water cos I'd wash my hands because they feel itchy but then 'success', so I'm smiling.

The citric disrupts any clear sense of boundaries between the 'real' (ontological) and 'known' (epistemological) event. It acts to both constitute and know the 'success' as inextricably bound. The drugs, heroin and crack cocaine, are also drawn (in brown, centre), but perhaps in a less marked way than the syringe (in red, centre-left), or cooker (in green, centre-left). I highlight these substances and 'things' here to show the many nonhuman bodies involved in the injecting event that get noticed through these drawings.

Moreover, the body mapping captured a sense of muddle and uncertainty in the event, where things seem to suddenly come together (or, as one participant put it, 'it will just happen'), but can just as easily shift, and fall apart (or 'drop over' as Lucy puts it above). Highlighting this fragility further, Lucy says 'there's this 50/50 if it's going to work: 50 heaven/50 hell'. However, this is not to suggest a lack of agency, just a different kind. Following Annemarie Mol:

> Once it is singled out as a topic of study, even undergoing appears to have little to do with being passive. It is hard work. Ask amateurs – of music, *of drugs*, of wine – and follow what they do in practice. They do a lot: their pleasure depends on preparations. (Mol, 2010, p. 256, my emphasis)

The collaborative 'success' of the injection is based on a finely attuned balancing act of bodies, so to assume Lucy and other participants a hierarchically more active role than their nonhuman partners (mastery over their tools/environment) would be to underplay their coproduction. Accordingly, the 'success' of the injecting event was permanently at risk or 'on the tilt' and required, to extend Lucy's metaphor, constant work to 'keep it upright'.

One participant, Simon, illuminates some of this work.

> Now, what I tend to do. It has to be when I'm ... it'd have to be in the evening. I will have to have eaten. I'd have to have had a few drinks to relax me, definitely will have to have eaten. I mean, you know, I used to do it in the morning before I'd even woken up kind of thing, you know what I mean, so I would have had no blood pressure what so ever. But because my veins were so good it would still work. Now that, no way, it has to be the whole thing of hot water, do the washing up, make sure I've eaten and you can see the little tiny marks. So what it is now, is that I'll see a tiny little one, or I'll just do it by feeling, you just rub very, very, very gently, rubbing your hand around like that (rubs his hand delicately), and I'll just feel something that gives a little bit and I know that's a vein.

The timings for when Simon injects are important. It has to be in the evening. He has to have had something to eat and drink. He has to increase his heart rate to raise a vein. Other participants talked about exercising, such as fast cycling, to stimulate the venal system. Simon also mentions 'the whole thing of hot water', that is, he explains, he does the washing-up so that the hot water and activity helps a vein to swell and make itself visible and viable. He then performs the delicate operation of feeling his hand for a slight change in texture and give in a vein which indicates there is blood and the vein is large enough to hold the needle steady without piercing through the other side causing a 'miss hit'. The *success* of the injection is reliant on all these practices – to make something happen, or 'occur', to use Gomart and Hennion's (1999) term. But where Gomart and Hennion suggest a 'passing' – what might be called 'mediation' in other ANT accounts of drug use – between 'subjects and objects', 'control and loss of control', 'the body and the head', I feel this is incongruent with the shared agencies expressed here, where the divisions were never so clear cut and the points of seizure were already co-produced. In other words, the connections shown above were only ever partial, in a process of 'staying upright'. Or, to follow Deleuze (1993), the event is only ever 'happening'.

In this sense, whether, how, and to what ends an injection of heroin and/or crack cocaine has an effect was far from chosen. With the individual entangled in the event, it depended on the coming together of an assembly of heterogeneous bodies, human and nonhuman, made possible through an equally complicated set of techno-corporeal preparatory practices. Thus, participants expressed an intra-corporeality, that is, an emergent embodiment of human and nonhuman processes. This is perhaps also where the events perspective most departs from earlier attempts to go beyond the individual in notions of the 'risk environment' (noted in the introduction). Where the 'risk environment' takes contextual influences seriously through an appreciation of how social, economic, political and discursive structures *interact* with the human subject to result in harmful consequences, here, in reconfiguring the boundaries between the subject and object, inside and outside, and body and environment, I want to think about how the 'human' body itself comes into being through these injecting events. That is, how the injecting event produces more than affects and effects ('what occurs') as pleasurable, in coming together in 'successful' ways, and painful, in coming together in unsuccessful ways, but also the ways it produces new bodies ('what becomes').

Becoming-with drugs

> The posthuman condition urges us to think critically and creatively about who and what we are actually in the process of becoming. (Braidotti, 2013, p. 12)

So far, I have highlighted the injecting event as a fragile modality of connection, which goes beyond any one controlling or agentic component, instead, held together through a complex collaborative effort. This disrupts previous accounts of the rational individual in harm reduction and in other areas of sociology where, for example, the 'controlled loss of control' model has been prominent (see Poulsen, 2015). On the other hand, it also unsettles addiction narratives that centre on the power of the controlling, disempowering drug. In extending this account of the injecting event, I want to consider the various ways participants depict 'becoming-with drugs' (Michael & Rosengarten, 2012), which shifts corporeal boundaries yet further.

These points of transformation were felt both as stabilising (in becoming-normal, see Dennis, 2016b) and changing the self (in becoming-other). However, there is a fine line between the two as both are underpinned by process, that is, 'stabilising' should not be confused with anything static. This socio-material performativity is captured by one participant who says 'a lot of people want the up, the buzz as well, as lots of people go to work, working, living relatively normal lives, y'know, they have *things to keep together*'. Beyond the event itself, drugs can be seen here to play a wider role in 'keeping things together'. This is also described by another participant, Sandra, who depicts (Figure 2) the role of injecting heroin in enabling 'functioning for the rest of the day', 'shopping', and 'daily life'.

Sandra, who was 48 years old, and had been injecting heroin on and off for the past 25 years, spoke of how, like her friend Gwen (who I also spoke to), injecting heroin played an important role in not only enabling everyday activities but in easing her health problems.

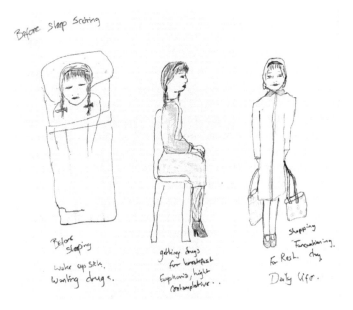

Figure 2. Sandra's body map.

> What happened is, me and Gwen both got the same thing, we've got COPD [Chronic Obstructive Pulmonary Disease], so we can't breathe without gear [heroin], it suppresses your breathing which really helps. We can't breathe without the gear. And also, I've got a degenerative back problem so I can't walk without it. I could not walk. *I couldn't walk at all.*

Gwen too tells me how heroin helps her to feel better. Or to appropriate Cameron Duff's Deleuzian notion of health, to become healthier. For Duff (2014), health is defined by one's capacity to affect and be affected, or 'power of acting'. Health, Duff says, 'may be understood to involve those forms of bodily activity that extend a body's range of action' (2014, p. 75). Drugs therefore, for some, in some instances, may contribute towards this power, which disrupts a dominant discourse on harm.

> At the moment I'm happy to carry on because I'm not very well anyway and it helps me. It helps me through the day, I can admit that I actually like doing it, because I'm having a miserable life with my illnesses. I've got Crohn's disease and the thing about Crohn's disease is that you have constant diarrhoea and pain, heroin and morphine constipates you so it stops the diarrhoea so I'm actually using it medicinally as well. They say that 'if we could pre-scribe you morphine for your condition we would but we're not allowed to'. (Gwen)

Furthermore, as Gwen hints to, in admitting 'I actually like doing it', becoming-with drugs does not only bring bodies together in a stabilising, normalising, or health-giving ways, but for some participants was intimately involved in *enhancing* life or becoming some*body* else. For example, participants talked about how drugs enabled them to become friendlier, more energetic, tolerant, and sociable. To this effect, Dimitri says:

> My mates say, when I haven't had nothing I'm quiet, and then as soon as I've had something I'm completely changed, my mood's like up, and I'm taking the piss and everything like that, complete, like you can spot it, you can, the complete change is like yeah, totally different.

Another participant depicted this change of self in drawing a picture of herself as superwoman, overtly signalling the role of drugs in making her into something more-than-human, with, she says, enhanced energy and tolerance of others.

However, as Peta Malins warns, through a reading of Deleuze's assemblage:

> Within each drug assemblage, the body connects up not only to the drug (its texture, its smell, its taste, its appear-ance, its speed) but also to other bodies and machines – people, substances, knowledges, institutions – any of which may redirect or block its flows of desire. (2004, p. 89)

Therefore, becoming-with drugs was not only life sustaining and enhancing, but could also be con-straining or containing, in particular, when connecting with bodies that have 'stratifying tendencies'. In Deleuze and Guattari's words:

> *Strata* are Layers, Belts. They consist of giving form to matters, or imprisoning intensities or locking singularities into systems of resonance and redundancy, of producing upon the body of the earth molecules large and small and organising them into molar aggregates. (2004, p. 45)

Participants give vivid accounts of how, in being linked up to, to use Malins's phrase, the 'junkie image', and the syringe, especially, they were constrained in these ways: prevented from becoming 'legitimate', 'worthy' or 'trusted' patients, friends, daughters, employees, customers etc. These shifts in boundaries get exemplified in Lucy's recount of an incident in which her boyfriend's step-mother found their disused syringes. He 'was wacked around the face' and 'we were told that we should have labels put on us saying that we're dirty junkies'. As these connections to the syringe were not visible, the step-mother, in her rage, demands that they should where a sign to literally transfix or 'lock' (to use Deleuze & Guattari's words above) the 'junkie' identity and block other ways of becoming, such as, one can guess, being able to walk down the street unnoticed, get a job, etc.

Through this analysis, it appears that drugs do not have innate qualities but can be part of good and bad encounters (Keane, 2003) as bodily boundaries shift capacities to affect and be affected. That is, 'good' when linked up with bodies to become 'healthier' or somehow better than themselves (increas-ing capacities to act), and 'bad' when linked to bodies with stratifying tendencies, which tie bodies down and constrain them (decreasing capacities to act). In prioritising the event over forms or bodies as given, that is, in considering how bodily forms *come into being through the event* – in connecting to other bodies – harm reduction is required to shift its focus beyond the human. Where a 'social science for harm reduction' has already been influential in decentring 'the individual' with the 'situated individual' and 'risk environment', the analysis here suggests a further step is needed towards what could be considered individuals-*as*-situations.

Harm reduction beyond the human: what does this look like in practice?

In moving away from 'the human' towards *becoming through events* we can start to think about harm reduction in more open ways. I will now think about what this might look like in practice. First, as we have seen, 'events' are uncertain, fragile and precarious, and thus they invoke a need for *contingency* over fixed solutions based on causes and effects. Indeed, rigid policies and interventions could be 'blocking' rather than enabling ways of becoming-other. Second, by understanding subject formation as 'event-full', this requires 'response-ability' (Barad, 2012; Haraway, 2008) in research and policy to attend to and bring into being more *careful* forms (Martin, Myers, & Viseu, 2015; Puig de la Bellacasa, 2011). We must learn to attune to these different forms and what they can tell us about the world, as well as being accountable for what gets made, in order to bring bodies together in 'healthier' ways.

A call for contingency in drug treatment policy and practice is arguably already one of harm reduction's biggest strengths. As we saw in the abstract, harm reduction is built on accepting that people will use drugs (accepting these attachments, if you like) and, rather than judging or moralising, working with these encounters to make them as safe as possible. Inspired by a notion of contingency, we can take these insights even further towards the level of relationality seen here, and the role of drug research and intervention in bringing about relationalities of new kinds. Drawing from Sara Ahmed:

> The word 'contingency' has the same root in Latin as the word 'contact' (Latin: contingere: com-, with; tangere, to touch). Contingency is linked then to proximity, to getting close enough to touch another and to be moved by another. (2004, p. 28)

Contingency incites an awareness to our existence in terms of the *outside within* as seen in the accounts of drug-body relations. Therefore, in light of the event, it is perhaps no surprise that when I asked one participant, Mya, about why she continued using drugs, she replied:

> *And the way of life.* You know, how can I get a methadone script when I'm not living nowhere, how can I get a doctor when I can't give no address. From when you're homeless, everything is against you. You can't get a doctor, you can't get a prescription, there's no way out. So you just go deeper and deeper into it.

It is not only in connection to drugs that she goes 'deeper and deeper into it' or experiences addiction (blocked ways of becoming-other) but in these connections with other bodies – 'the way of life' – including the legal system, institutions, knowledges and policies, which means she has no housing, doctor or prescription for an opiate substitute. Therefore, drug treatment systems that make it harder for contingency, that resist relationality or fail to be 'in touch', like making it difficult to access methadone outside 'working hours', could actually be blocking ways of becoming-other.

As well as contingency being needed within the administration of opiate substitution treatment (e.g. Fraser & Valentine, 2008; Harris & Rhodes, 2013), like other harm reduction technologies (e.g. Bourgois, 2000), for many participants, contingency was also required in the substances or technologies themselves. For Tom, buprenorphine, an opiate agonist and antagonist, did not have such contingency. Instead, where the agonist component or 'blocker' failed and he 'found' (a word that emphasises the workings of an event rather than an individual) himself using heroin 'on top' of his prescription he entered into precipitated withdrawals.

> Years ago I had terrible troubles with Subutex (brand name for buprenorphine). I sort of went to get clean, got down to about 10 mil of methadone and then went onto buprenorphine cos it's got the blocker [antagonist] in it supposedly [...] But I found the transition horrible, and then I found out that the blocker only works for about 4 hours so then, when I found myself using on top, I found it fucking murder. Switching to buprenorphine, I found it really hard. It just ended up being a waste of a script. I think methadone is much easier.

For Tom, methadone, an opiate agonist, allowed for these moments when the drug assemblage might take him, where buprenorphine could not ('you couldn't use on top'), meaning that when he did, the script 'ended up being a waste', and he went back to exclusively using heroin. For Tom, methadone has more contingency, it is more 'in-touch' with these assemblic moments, or sudden *eventful* coming togethers of bodies in which he 'found [himself] using'. This adds weight to similar calls for 'convenience' in harm reduction (Fraser, 2013).

Therefore, to return to Keane's (2003) reading of Stengers mentioned at the beginning, 'rather than promoting [human] freedom as a moral principle or universal ideal', Keane 'focuses attention on the effect of different programmes and campaigns on individuals' capacity for freedom and ethical self-formation' (p. 231). This can be seen to move the ethics of harm reduction as a matter of fact – based on the human – to what Latour (2004) would call a 'matter of concern' – where what constitutes harm (impingements to freedom and self-formation) is open to iterative debate and different programmes. Critical attention is shifted from the principle of the programme to its effects or 'what occurs'.

However, thinking about how bodies become through events perhaps turns harm reduction research and practice as a 'matter of concern', or matter of 'what occurs', made up of a negotiated apparatus beyond the human, into what Puig de la Bellacasa (2011) calls a 'matter of care', or what I have suggested can be seen as an added concern for 'what becomes'. 'We must take care of things in order to remain responsible for their becomings' (Puig de la Bellacasa, 2011, p. 90), and therefore we must be accountable for what gets made in research and practice alike, and the bodily boundaries we inevitably bring into being. As seen here, in opening up boundaries beyond the human, we can account for the many ways, including positive ways bodies become-with drugs.

I have suggested that one way care might be brought into our research is through the notion of 'touch'. Ahmed and Barad, like Puig de la Bellacasa, all draw on 'touch' to stress these collective ways of knowing and engaging with the world – to touch and 'to be in touch' is to be attuned and responsive to these different forms. For example, many drug worker accounts highlighted the need for 'intuition' and 'creativity' over protocol in order to cope with the multiple ways bodies become through injecting or drug events and thus the different ways to make them 'healthier', to use Duff's notion. For some participants, like Gwen, Sandra and Mya, this may include the continued use of opiates. Therefore, instead of favouring increasingly punitive measures (e.g. Wintour, 2015), based on assumed effects of drugs as bad, we need to increase awareness, tolerance and responsiveness to the event in order to learn from and be part of making bodies in new and better ways.

Conclusion

> The ethical imagination is alive and well in posthuman subjects, in the form of ontological relationality. A sustainable ethics for non-unitary subjects rests on an enlarged sense of inter-connection between self and others, including the non-human. (Braidotti, 2013, p. 190)

Responding to shifts within the social sciences of drug use, this paper has tried to move us yet further away from the human or individual, that is, even in its strategic or situated forms, towards what are potentially more ethical posthuman injecting or drug-using collectives. By exploring injecting events as connections of bodies, substances, images and things in participants' accounts of becoming-with drugs, not only is the heterogeneity and fragility of the event highlighted, but also what participants are actually in the process of becoming. Where some injecting events enabled positively felt experiences and subjectivities, other events – connecting with bodies with stratifying tendencies such as the syringe – materialised in negative ways, blocking ways of becoming-other. Indeed, drug treatment services were sometimes part of these formations. This calls for a more 'response-*able*' approach to drug use. To appropriate Puig de la Bellacasa words, we need to be aware and care for these events in order 'to remain responsible for their becomings'. Consequently, I argue that two such possibilities for a harm reduction in light of our posthumanism lie in the practices of contingency and care. Building contingency into our technologies and practices means we can allow for the ambiguities, differences and uncertainties intrinsic to the complexities of drug events and what becomes. In caring, we must act to increase our capacities to be affected by these events, to be part of increasing good affects ('power of acting' in becoming-other), as well as decreasing the potential for bad affects (blocked becomings).

It is in this sense that we, in drug research, policy and practice, can most intimately be part of making bodies better.

Acknowledgements

I am hugely thankful to everybody who generously agreed to participate in this study. I would also like to thank my supervisors, Magdalena Harris and Tim Rhodes, for their support, Suzanne Fraser, for her useful feedback on earlier iterations of the paper, and the two anonymous reviewers for their helpful suggestions.

Disclosure statement

No potential conflict of interest was reported by the author.

Funding

This research was undertaken at the London School of Hygiene & Tropical Medicine, with the support of a 4-year PhD studentship from the Economic and Social Research Council.

References

Ahmed, S. (2004). *The cultural politics of emotion*. Edinburgh: Edinburgh University Press.

Barad, K. (2007). *Meeting the universe halfway: Quantum physics and the entanglement of matter and meaning*. Durham, NC: Duke University Press.

Barad, K. (2012). On touching: The inhuman that therefore I am. *Differences: A Journal of Feminist Cultural Studies, 23*, 206–223. doi:10.1215/10407391-1892943

Bergschmidt, V. B. (2004). Pleasure, power and dangerous substances: Applying Foucault to the study of 'heroin dependence' in Germany. *Anthropology and Medicine, 11*, 59–73. doi:10.1080/1364847042000204915

Bøhling, F. (2014). Crowded contexts: On the affective dynamics of alcohol and other drug use in nightlife spaces. *Contemporary Drug Problems, 41*, 361–392. doi:10.1177/009145091404100305

Bourgois, P. (2000). Disciplining addictions: The bio-politics of methadone and heroin in the United States. *Culture, Medicine & Psychiatry, 24*, 165–195. doi:10.1023/A:1005574918294

Braidotti, R. (2013). *The posthuman*. Cambridge: Polity Press.

Crawford, A. (2010). If 'the body keeps the score': Mapping the dissociated body in trauma narrative, intervention, and theory. *University of Toronto Quarterly, 79*, 702–719. doi:10.1353/utq.2010.0231

Deleuze, G. (1990). *The logic of sense*. New York, NY: Columbia University Press.

Deleuze, G. (1993). *The fold: Leibniz and the Baroque*. London: Bloomsbury.

Deleuze, G. (2004). *Difference and repetition*. London: Bloomsbury.

Deleuze, G., & Guattari, F. (2004). *A thousand plateaus: Capitalism and schizophrenia*. London: Continuum.

Demant, J. (2009). When alcohol acts: An Actor-network approach to teenagers, alcohol and parties. *Body & Society, 15*, 25–46. doi:10.1177/1357034x08100145

Dennis, F. (2016a). Encountering "Triggers": Drug-body-world entanglements of injecting drug use. *Contemporary Drug Problems, 43*, 126–141. doi:10.1177/0091450916636379

Dennis, F. (2016b). Drugs: Bodies becoming "normal". *M/C Journal*. Retrieved from http://journal.media-culture.org.au/index.php/mcjournal/article/view/1073

Dilkes-Frayne, E. (2014). Tracing the "Event" of drug use: "Context" and the coproduction of a night out on MDMA. *Contemporary Drug Problems, 41*, 445–479. doi:10.1177/009145091404100308

Duff, C. (2007). Towards a theory of drug use contexts: Space, embodiment and practice. *Addiction Research & Theory, 15*, 503–519. doi:10.1080/16066350601165448

Duff, C. (2012). Accounting for context: Exploring the role of objects and spaces in the consumption of alcohol and other drugs. *Social & Cultural Geography, 13*, 145–159. doi:10.1080/14649365.2012.655765

Duff, C. (2013). The social life of drugs. *International Journal of Drug Policy, 24*, 167–172. doi:10.1016/j.drugpo.2012.12.009

Duff, C. (2014). *Assemblages of health: Deleuze's empiricism and the ethology of life*. New York, NY: Springer.

Duff, C. (2016). Assemblages, territories, contexts. *International Journal of Drug Policy, 33*, 15–20. doi:10.1016/j.drugpo.2015.10.003

Dwyer, R., Fraser, S., & Treloar, C. (2011). Doing things together? Analysis of health education materials to inform hepatitis C prevention among couples. *Addiction Research and Theory, 19*, 352–361. doi:10.3109/16066359.2011.562619

Erickson, P., Riley, D., Cheung, Y., & O'Hare, P. (1997). *Harm reduction: A new direction for drug policies and programs*. Toronto: University of Toronto Press.

Ezard, N. (2001). Public health, human rights and the harm reduction paradigm: From risk reduction to vulnerability reduction. *International Journal of Drug Policy, 12*, 207–219. doi:10.1016/S0955-3959(01)00093-7

Farrugia, A. (2015). 'You can't just give your best mate a massive hug every day': young men, play and MDMA. *Contemporary Drug Problems, 42*, 240–256. doi:10.1177/0091450915601520

Fraser, M. (2011). Facts, ethics and event. In C. Bruun Jensen & K. Rödje (Eds.), *Deleuzian intersections: Science, technology, anthropology* (pp. 55–83). Oxford, New York: Berghahn Books.

Fraser, S. (2004). 'It's your life!': Injecting drug users, individual responsibility and hepatitis C prevention. *Health: An Interdisciplinary Journal for the Social Study of Health, Illness and Medicine, 8*, 199–221. doi:10.1177/1363459304041070

Fraser, S. (2006). The chronotope of the queue: Methadone maintenance treatment and the production of time, space and subjects. *International Journal of Drug Policy, 17*, 192–202. doi:10.1016/j.drugpo.2006.02.010

Fraser, S. (2013). The missing mass of morality: A new fitpack design for hepatitis C prevention in sexual partnerships. *International Journal of Drug Policy, 24*, 212–219. doi:10.1016/j.drugpo.2013.03.009

Fraser, S., Rance, J., & Treloar, C. (2016). Hepatitis C prevention and convenience: Why do people who inject drugs in sexual partnerships 'run out' of sterile equipment? *Critical Public Health, 26*, 294–306. doi:10.1080/09581596.2015.1036839

Fraser, S., & Seear, K. (2011). *Making disease, making citizens: The politics of hepatitis C.* Farnham: Ashgate.

Fraser, S., Treloar, C., Bryant, J., & Rhodes, T. (2014). Hepatitis C prevention education needs to be grounded in social relationships. *Drugs: Education, Prevention and Policy, 21*, 88–92. doi:10.3109/09687637.2013.776517

Fraser, S., & Valentine, K. (2006). 'Making blood flow': Materializing blood in body modification and blood-borne virus prevention. *Body & Society, 12*, 97–119. doi:10.1177/1357034x06061191

Fraser, S., & Valentine, K. (2008). *Substance and substitution: Methadone subjects in liberal societies.* Basingstoke: Palgrave Macmillan.

Gomart, E., & Hennion, A. (1999). A sociology of attachment: Music amateurs, drug users. In J. Law & J. Hassard (Eds.), *Actor network theory and after* (pp. 220–248). Oxford: Blackwell/Sociological Review.

Haraway, D. J. (2008). *When species meet.* Minneapolis: University of Minnesota Press.

Harris, M., & Rhodes, T. (2013). Methadone diversion as a protective strategy: The harm reduction potential of 'generous constraints'. *International Journal of Drug Policy, 24*, e43–e50. doi:10.1016/j.drugpo.2012.10.003

Hathaway, A. D. (2001). Shortcomings of harm reduction: Toward a morally invested drug reform strategy. *International Journal of Drug Policy, 12*, 125–137. doi:10.1016/S0955-3959(01)00085-8

Heather, N., Wodak, A., Nadelmann, E., & O'Hare, P. (Eds.). (1993). *Psychoactive drugs and harm reduction: From faith to science.* London: Whurr.

Hunt, N. (2004). Public health or human rights: What comes first? *International Journal of Drug Policy, 15*, 231–237. doi:10.1016/j.drugpo.2004.02.001

Jürgens, R. J., Csete, J. J., Amon, S., Baral, C., & Beyrer, C. (2010). People who use drugs, HIV, and human rights. *The Lancet, 376*, 475–485. doi:10.1016/S0140-6736(10)60830-6

Keane, H. (2003). Critiques of harm reduction, morality and the promise of human rights. *International Journal of Drug Policy, 14*, 227–232. doi:10.1016/S0955-3959(02)00151-2

Kerr, T., Wood, E., Betteridge, G., Lines, R., & Jürgens, R. (2004). Harm reduction in prisons: A 'rights based analysis'. *Critical Public Health, 14*, 1–16. doi:10.1080/09581590400027478

Latour, B. (2004). Why has critique run out of steam? From matters of fact to matters of concern. *Critical Inquiry, 30*, 225–248. doi:10.1086/421123

Lury, C., & Wakeford, N. (2012). *Inventive methods: The happening of the social.* London: Routledge.

Malinowska-Sempruch, K., & Gallagher, S. (Eds.). (2004). *War on drugs, HIV/AIDS and human rights.* New York, NY: The International Debate Education Association.

Malins, P. (2004). Machinic assemblages: Deleuze, Guattari and an ethico-aesthetics of drug use. *Janus Head, 7*, 84–104. Retrieved from http://www.janushead.org/7-1/malins.pdf

Martin, A., Myers, N., & Viseu, A. (2015). The politics of care in technoscience. *Social Studies of Science, 45*, 625–641. doi:10.1177/0306312715602073

McLean, K. (2011). The biopolitics of needle exchange in the United States. *Critical Public Health, 21*, 71–79. doi:10.1080/09581591003653124

Michael, M. (2015). Ignorance and the epistemic choreography of method. In M. Gross & L. McGoey (Eds.), *Routledge International Handbook of Ignorance Studies* (pp. 84–92). London: Routledge, Taylor & Francis Group.

Michael, M., & Rosengarten, M. (2012). Medicine: Experimentation, politics, emergent bodies. *Body & Society, 18*, 1–17. doi:10.1177/1357034X12451860

Miller, P. G. (2001). A critical review of the harm minimization ideology in Australia. *Critical Public Health, 11*, 167–178. doi:10.1080/09581590110039865

Mol, A. (2010). Actor-network theory: Sensitive terms and enduring tensions. *Kölner Zeitschrift für Soziologie und Sozialpsychologie, 50*, 253–269. Retrieved from http://dare.uva.nl/document/2/90295

Moore, D., & Fraser, S. (2006). Putting at risk what we know: Reflecting on the drug-using subject in harm reduction and its political implications. *Social Science & Medicine, 62*, 3035–3047. doi:10.1016/j.socscimed.2005.11.067

Mugford, S. (1993). Harm reduction: Does it lead where its proponents imagine? In N. Heather, A. Wodak, E. Nadelmann, & P. O'Hare (Eds.), *Psychoactive drugs and harm reduction: From faith to science* (pp. 21–34). London: Whurr.

O'Hare, P., Newcombe, R., Matthews, A., Buning, E., & Drucker, E. (Eds.). (1991). *The reduction of drug-related harm*. London: Routledge.

O'Malley, P., & Valverde, M. (2004). Pleasure, freedom and drugs: The uses of 'pleasure' in liberal governance of drug and alcohol consumption. *Sociology, 38*, 25–42. doi:10.1177/0038038504039359

Poulsen, M. (2015). Embodied subjectivities: Bodily subjectivity and changing boundaries in post-human alcohol practices. *Contemporary Drug Problems, 42*, 3–19. doi:10.1177/0091450915569499

Puig de la Bellacasa, M. (2011). Matters of care in technoscience: Assembling neglected things. *Social Studies of Science, 41*, 85–106. doi:10.1177/0306312710380301

Race, K. (2014). Complex events: Drug effects and emergent causality. *Contemporary Drug Problems, 41*, 301–334. doi:10.1177/009145091404100303

Race, K. (2015). 'Party and Play': Online hook-up devices and the emergence of PNP practices among gay men. *Sexualities, 18*, 253–275. doi:10.1177/1363460714550913

Release. (2016). *Drug policy in the UK and its intersection with international human rights*. Submission to the office of the high commissioner for human rights from Release. Retrieved from http://www.release.org.uk/sites/default/files/pdf/publications/Release%20submision%20on%20drug%20policy%20in%20the%20UK%20-%20OHCHR%20final.pdf

Rhodes, T. (2002). The 'risk environment': A framework for understanding and reducing drug-related harm. *International Journal of Drug Policy, 13*, 85–94. doi:10.1016/S0955-3959(02)00007-5

Rhodes, T. (2009). Risk environments and drug harms: A social science for harm reduction approach. *International Journal of Drug Policy, 20*, 193–201. doi:10.1016/j.drugpo.2008.10.003

Rhodes, T., Singer, M., Bourgois, P., Friedman, S. R., & Strathdee, S. A. (2005). The social structural production of HIV risk among injecting drug users. *Social Science & Medicine, 61*, 1026–1044. doi:10.1016/j.socscimed.2004.12.024

Rumbold, G., Kellehear, A., & Hamilton, M. (Eds.). (1998). *Drug use in Australia: A harm minimisation approach*. Oxford: Oxford University Press.

Seear, K., & Moore, D. (2014). Complexity: Researching alcohol and other drugs in a multiple world. *Contemporary Drug Problems, 41*, 295–300. doi:10.1177/009145091404100302

Stagoll, C. (2010). Event. In A. Parr (Ed.), *The Deleuze dictionary* (revised ed., pp. 89–91). Edinburgh: Edinburgh University Press.

Stengers, I., & Ralet, O. (1997). Drugs: Ethical choice or moral consensus. In I. Stengers (Ed.), *Power and invention: Situating science* (pp. 215–232). Minneapolis: University of Minnesota Press.

Stevens, A. (2011). Drug policy, harm and human rights: A rationalist approach. *International Journal of Drug Policy, 22*, 233–238. doi:10.1016/j.drugpo.2011.02.003

Tarr, J., & Thomas, H. (2011). Mapping embodiment: Methodologies for representing pain and injury. *Qualitative Research, 11*, 141–157. doi:10.1177/1468794110394067

UNAIDS. (2015). *Do no harm: Health, human rights and people who use drugs*. Retrieved from http://www.unaids.org/sites/default/files/media_asset/donoharm_en.pdf

Vargas, E. V. (2010). Tarde on drugs, or measure against suicide. In M. Candea (Ed.), *The social after Gabriel Tarde: Debates and assessments* (pp. 208–230). London: Routledge.

Wintour, P. (2015, July 29). Obese people and drug users who refuse treatment could have benefits cut. *The Guardian*. Retrieved from http://www.theguardian.com/society/2015/jul/29/benefits-drugs-alcohol-obesity-refusing-treatment-review

Biopolitical precarity in the permeable body: the social lives of people, viruses and their medicines

Elizabeth Mills

ABSTRACT

This article is based on multi-sited ethnography that traced a dynamic network of actors (activists, policy-makers, health care systems, pharmaceutical companies) and actants (viruses and medicines) that shaped South African women's access to, and embodiment of, antiretroviral therapies (ARVs). Using actor network theory and post-humanist performativity as conceptual tools, the article explores how bodies become the meeting place for HIV and ARVs, or non-human actants. The findings centre around two linked sets of narratives that draw the focus out from the body to situate the body in relation to South Africa's shifting biopolitical landscape. The first set of narratives articulate how people perceive the intra-action of HIV and ARVs in their sustained vitality. The second set of narratives articulate the complex embodiment of these actants as a form biopolitical precarity. These narratives flow into each other and do not represent a totalising view of the effects of HIV and ARVs in the lives of the people with whom I worked. The positive effects of ARVs (as unequivocally essential for sustaining life) were implicit and the precarious vitality of the people in this ethnography was fundamental. However, a related and emergent set of struggles become salient during the study that complicate a view of ARVs as a 'technofix'. These emergent struggles were biopolitical, and they related first to the intra-action of HIV and ARVs 'within' the body; and second, to the 'outside' socio-economic context in which people's bodies were situated.

In the wake of the struggle for antiretrovirals in South Africa

President Zuma's face smiled down from a large billboard, impressing his vision for South Africa onto throngs of jetlagged people as we navigated our bodies and luggage trolleys out of Cape Town's International Airport. The billboard emphasised the government's commitment to creating decent jobs, education, health, fighting crime and rural development. I manoeuvred my luggage under the billboard and into the car.

With Khayelitsha behind me and Table Mountain in front of me, I drove past the green mosque that marked the turn-off to Nyanga – Khayelitsha's neighboring township and my fieldsite in 2003 and 2004. In the course of my ethnography with Luvuyolwethu, an HIV home-based care organisation, I came to know Nyanga's streets as I walked from one home to another with the carers during their 'rounds'. This is how I met Peggy. She lived with her 22-year-old son, Zithulele, and her 25-year-old daughter, Patricia. When I started my fieldwork, Patricia was still able to sit up in the bed that Luvuyolwethu had set up in the sitting area of Peggy's home. Without antiretrovirals (ARVs), HIV had become AIDS and Patricia had become immobile. We did not realise – or perhaps articulate – that when we moved Patricia from her bed to lie down in the back seat of my car, eventually to lie down in Groote Schuur hospital, that she would not come back home. We went to visit Patricia a few days later: on the cusp of death, she had been heavily sedated with morphine. After driving in silence most of the way back home, Peggy pulled her jersey more tightly around her body and said, 'I fought in the streets for this government. Now the holes in my roof are just bigger and they are not giving me medicine for my daughter'. Patricia died three days later, just a month before the government was forced by cabinet to initiate the ARV roll-out.

At that time, in 2003, the presence of the post-apartheid state in people's lives was felt through its absence, embodied in death, evident in the blossoming of wooden crosses on graves carefully dug to run as closely as possible alongside each other. In the course of my fieldwork, the graves had pushed out and against the feeble fence that lined N1 – the main road that ran like Nyanga's spine between this space of death and homes of Luvuyolwethu's clients. On a bitterly cold winter's day, Peggy's family and I clustered around the parcel of earth that had been designated as Patricia's grave. When we returned from Patricia's funeral to Peggy's home, we all washed our hands in one of the three buckets that had been placed in her front yard. Peggy explained to me that by washing our hands after Patricia's burial we signified to the ancestors that we had distanced ourselves from death and looked, instead, towards life.

In this pre-ARV era, HIV became AIDS became death so rapidly that the forward slash between HIV/AIDS made sense. In 2016, it no longer does. ARVs have pried open the space between HIV and AIDS. Now, this opening out of life brings to light a set of complex challenges around the biopolitics of HIV therapies and the socio-economic conditions in which life on ARVs is lived. These new generation struggles call into focus an assemblage of actants and actors that, together, are networked into women's embodied precarity. While a longer life with HIV is possible through 'technologies of life' like ARVs, for the women I worked with over a decade I met Peggy and Patricia, it is still a precarious life that, everyday, pushes out and against the possibility of death.

This article draws on ethnographic research conducted in South Africa between 2010 and 2011. Through this research, I explored two interlinked themes: first, women's embodied experience of HIV and ARVs and, second, women's perception of and engagement with the state based on their embodied experience of illness and biomedicine. Their conjunction is explored through the concept of 'biopolitical precarity'. Drawing on post-humanist performativity as a conceptual tool (Barad, 2003, 2007), the article traces the 'intra-action' of HIV and ARVs as non-human actants (Latour, 2005) inside the body, and it locates the body in a broader context where emergent biomedical and socio-economic challenges confound a straightforward reading of ARVs as the solution to the problem of HIV.

Ethno-theoretical connections

[E]thnographic engagement can help us chart some of the complex and often contradictory ways in which neo-liberalizing health structures, moral economy, and biology are forged in local worlds where biotechnology and structural violence now exist side-by-side. (Biehl, 2004, p. 125)

In researching the embodied ramifications of illness and medicine on people's perception of the state, the men and women I met during my fieldwork took the feminist adage that the personal is political and mixed it up, thoroughly. The ethnography called for theoretical agility as people's accounts of the pathways that brought HIV and later ARVs as actants into their bodies implicated a network of actors, including scientists capable of reverse engineering essential HIV medicines in India's laboratories, South Africa's capacity to negotiate international trade law to access these medicines, (neoliberalising) health systems and its professionals who dispense medicines through small 'ARV-only' pharmaceutical counters in Khayelitsha's clinics. As I discuss in this article, my ethnographic research highlighted the importance of understanding the body as permeable, as neither material nor semiotic, but as a material-semiotic assemblage of networks.

My own thinking about HIV and ARVs as non-human actants follows the trajectory of thought around the social lives of things (Appadurai, 1988) and Whyte (2009) exploration of biomedicine as material medica. More recently, Michael and Rosengarten (2012) have looked at HIV prevention technologies, or pre-exposure prophylaxis (PrEP) as actants enmeshed in a web of relations. They consider two case studies (of the AIDS clock and accounts of randomised control trials) and explore how their 'global reach weaves into various local contingencies, particularly localizing critiques that emphasize the conditions of infection and death, and local political protest against the clinical trials' (2012, p. 95). As the work of these scholars suggest, globalisation and technological developments have certainly prompted a rethinking of governance in which we recognise that the contemporary 'body of the state' is far less 'sovereign' and far more porous than it was – ontologically and epistemologically – at the time of Weber (1984), Arendt (1958) and Foucault's (1978) theorising. Not only are the state and citizen porously implicated in each other's vitality but their own lives form part of a much larger assemblage. The term 'global assemblage' was coined by Collier and Ong (2005) to capture this dynamic, and has been used to reflect on the conflicts and controversies of globalisation, as changes in technologies, bodies and governments precipitated and were precipitated by global–local transformations.

At the same time that Collier and Ong (2005) coined 'global assemblage' for a collection of articles on the anthropology of ethics and technologies, George Marcus and Erkan Sarka were also, but more cynically, writing about the usefulness of this concept.

> While not one of the prime or key terms of recent and past discourses of theory in the social sciences … assemblage in its uses here and there is actually keenly symptomatic of one of the major, if not the major, thrust of critical social and cultural theory toward the emphasis on the modernist focusing of attention on the always-emergent conditions of the present. (2006, pp. 101, 102)

I follow Marcus and Sarka's (2006) caution against an 'unthinking' application of assemblage by engaging with the tools offered through Actor Network Theory (ANT) to look at how assemblages take shape in people's lives. In line with Latour's (2005) assertion that we cannot simply look at the form that networks take, but need also to look at the associations that bring these elements together, Collier (2009) similarly argues – specifically in relation to the evolution of governmentality in Foucault's lectures – that we cannot only identify a form of the assemblage but that we need to extend our analysis to understand how this formation comes to take shape.

Assemblages and actor networks are not only conceptually useful, but they are also politically important: in using them together, they work against isolating politics from the body, and offer a set of tools to think usefully about the ways that actants and actors across scale, from the global to the molecular, are networked into an assemblage around the biopolitics of life. In this article, I use ANT to think about the actors (people and institutions) and non-human actants (HIV and ARVs) and how they interacted with each other through an assemblage that moved from under the skin right into the global arena of pharmaceutical developments, emerging trade policies and contested intellectual property rights.

In exploring the body as porously networked, I engage with medical anthropological approaches to biosocialities, and draw on the work of queer, feminist and science scholars who have similarly issued a challenge to representationalism. Responding to the assertion by medical anthropologists similarly researching ARV programmes in Sub-Saharan Africa that 'biosociality does not look inward to the body, but outward to human relationships' (Marsland, 2012, p. 473), this article suggests that perhaps there is a way of thinking about biosociality that does not ask us to look either into the body, or outward to socialities, but across them. To this end, this article juxtaposes interiority with ethnology: it looks across the world 'inside' and the world 'outside' the body.

'Diffractively reading the insights of feminist and queer theory and science studies approaches through one another entails thinking the "social" and the "scientific" together in an illuminating way' (Barad, 2003, p. 803). Building on insights from Butler (2004), Foucault (1978), Hacking (1990) and others, Barad (2007) issues a challenge to the metaphysical foundations of representationalism. She does by offering a radical post-humanist performative account of the relationship between material and discursive practices. A post-human account is one that makes explicit the implicit workings of humanist ideology that relies on the reification of 'the human' (and particularly the male human) (Braidotti, 2013, 2016). A post-humanist performative account is one that

> incorporates important material and discursive, social and scientific, human and nonhuman, and natural and cultural factors. A posthumanist account calls into question the givenness of the differential categories of 'human' and 'nonhuman,' examining the practices through which these differential boundaries are stabilized and destabilized. (Barad, 2003, p. 808)

This article integrates the conceptual approach of actor networks with post-humanist performativity to explore how bodies become the meeting place for HIV and ARVs, as non-human actants, and to trace how these actants disrupt distinctions or causal connections between the body they animate and the life they take on through this animation.

Butler (2009) and Haraway (1997) have also generated conceptual approaches that incorporate performativity in order to move away from representational accounts with regard to gender and science respectively. Performativity is defined as 'the citational practices which reproduce and/or subvert discourse and which enable and discipline subjects and their performances' (Gregson & Rose, 2000, p. 434). I draw on the notion of performativity, as distinct from but related to post-humanist performativity, to explore how individuals embody, reproduce and subvert discourse; and I use post-humanist performativity to draw the lives of ARVs and HIV as non-human actants into focus, as they simultaneously hold and generate a precarious vitality that transects the world 'inside' and the world 'outside' the body.

In place of 'interaction', I use the term 'intra-action' when discussing the lives of HIV and ARVs: the former reflects the Newtonian legacy in which 'things', or actants, are constructed as determinant, stable, prior-existing and bounded (Barad, 2003). Intra-action, instead, reflects this article's call for a material-semiotics that transcends the materiality of things (like medicines, bodies, viruses) and the discourses that shape them (like beliefs around health or practices of self-care) by showing their interconnections in an assemblage that is woven into people's bodies and lives.

Finally, I introduce the concept of 'biopolitical precarity' to denote the intra-action of actants that shape and are shaped by people's embodied experience of precarity in a biopolitical network that is threaded into the permeable body. I suggest that if we really are going to move beyond the 'nature/culture' dichotomy that separates biology from sociality we need to explore how the world 'outside' the body permeates and shapes life 'inside' the body. This requires a move away from privileging 'biology' as that which exists inside the body to recognising, through the concept of biopolitical precarity, how the body is porously networked into an assemblage that brings the 'outside' 'inside'.

A multi-sited ethnography

This article is based on a multi-sited ethnography conducted over 12 months in Khayelitsha, South Africa. Through this ethnography, I traced a dynamic network of actors (activists, policy-makers, health care systems, pharmaceutical companies) and actants (viruses and medicines) that shaped South African women's access to, and embodiment of, antiretroviral therapies (ARVs).

Khayelitsha is a semi-formal housing area in the Cape Town Metropole. In line with Loon's (2005) approach to the spatialisation of actants, actors and networks, my fieldwork similarly sought to trace a network of actors and actants as they were embodied by people living with HIV in this socially and politically dynamic space.

The space of Khayelitsha holds a history that reflects the South Africa's shifting biomedical and political landscapes: it was first place in South Africa where governmental and non-governmental actors worked together to provide ARVs. As people resumed their health, their testimonies about the Lazarus effect of these medicines further bolstered activists' calls for the government to roll out ARVs across the country (Robins, 2010). This particular confluence of history and space underpinned the rationale for conducting fieldwork in Khayelitsha.

The findings draw on ethnographic research with a core group of women on ARVs (aged 30–50); they all lived in Khayelitsha and had worked with Treatment Action Campaign (TAC) in the course of the decade long struggle for this treatment. In addition to participant observation, informal conversations and life history interviews, I used a set of visual research methods including participatory photography and film, and actor network mapping. The findings also reflect ethnographic research with a group of seven people with whom I have worked in various capacities since 2004. In this article, I reflect on ethnographic research conducted with this group in 2010 and 2010 in parallel with a series of body maps that they created in 2003 and 2011 (see: MacGregor, 2009). The 2011 body maps were created in a series of workshops, with the support of Jane Solomon, and they included a set of 'visual enquiries' that I proposed to the group (including creating an 'ARV timeline' and showing where they 'felt' medicine in the body). I then explored in greater detail through subsequent discussions with the artists.

I am aware that a visual and narrative approach to ethnography might re-create the very separation (between the body and mind, and between human and non-human actants) that this article speaks against. In order to address this limitation, I worked to interweave weave the main threads in my ethnography – narrative, visual and participant observation – together in order to ensure that I paid attention to silences and to embodied accounts that go beyond what is said, done or drawn.

The findings in this article corroborate the overall findings of the study that, in addition to participant observation, included: 20 key informant interviews with policy actors; 40 narrative life history interviews with men and women on ARVs; participant photography and film; and body and journey mapping.

Ethics permission for this study was formally obtained through the University of Sussex, through consent forms with each of the study participants, and through ongoing dialogue throughout the course of my research – beyond fieldwork – with the participants to discuss how they would like to be represented, which stories should be shared most boldly, and which stories should not be shared at all.

A shifting biopolitical landscape

The findings centre around two linked sets of narratives that draw the focus out from the body to situate the body in relation to South Africa's shifting biopolitical landscape. The first set of narratives articulate how people perceive the intra-action of HIV and ARVs in their sustained vitality. The second set of narratives articulate the complex embodiment of vitality alongside precarity. These narratives flow into each other and do not represent a totalising view of the effects of HIV and ARVs in the lives of the people with whom I worked.

The positive effects of ARVs (as unequivocally essential for sustaining life) were implicit and the precarious vitality of the people with whom I worked was fundamental. However, in the course my fieldwork, I found that a related and emergent set of struggles was becoming salient. They complicate the view that ARVs are a 'technofix' (Lock & Nguyen, 2010) and present a challenge to the idea that only 'local biologies' (Gilbert, 2013) like HIV and ARVs are embodied. As I go on to discuss, these emergent struggles were biopolitical, and they related first to the intra-action of HIV and ARVs 'within' the body; and second, to the 'outside' socio-economic context in which people's bodies were situated.

The struggle for ARVs and embodied vitality

In May, a week after the Municipal Elections, Mamello and I were walking down Queen Victoria street in central Cape Town. Not only did the name of the street speak to the colonial legacy of South Africa, but the Memorialised 'Slegs Blankes/Whites Only' bench that we passed outside the High Court was a reminder of South Africa's more recent history – one that Mamello had actively shaped through her affidavit and testimony in the court case that TAC brought against the government to compel them to provide PMTCT. We walked in silence past the bench; our conversations often had more silences than words.

Over months of walking and sometimes talking, I learnt that Mamello's activism was born from her anger with the government for failing to provide treatment to stop HIV from moving into her daughter's body. On this particular day, Mamello held up her thumb to me with its indelible stain, showing me that she had voted. I asked her why, and she pointed to Parliament, its white buildings barely visible over the green trees of the Company Gardens on Queen Victoria street. She said, 'I voted for my treatment'. She went on to say,

> I was here [gesturing to parliament] pressuring the government. I told them, 'You must give us the treatment because the people are dying'. The government – [former Health Minister] Manto Tshabalala-Msimang – was telling us that if we had HIV, we must take the veg… They ignored the virus. (Mamello, 2011 fieldwork notes)

I asked, 'When did they start taking things seriously?' 'As I give them pressure!' she replied. We turned right onto Wale Street and walked to the bottom of the stairs of the St George's Anglican Cathedral.

The Cathedral is situated next to the Parliament Buildings and has been used historically by apartheid and post-apartheid activists alike as a site of resistance and a place of mourning. It was, in fact, the same place where TAC had first assembled, almost 13 years previously. The Company Gardens, which move out from the Cathedral, mark an important politico-juridical intersection with the High Court on the right and Parliament on the left. It was through these two spaces of the state spanning policy development and juridical implementation that Mamello worked with TAC to challenge the pharmaceutical companies, and later the government, to provide ARVs to stop HIV from travelling through breastmilk and blood from a parent to their child, and through unprotected sex between people's bodies.

Zukile had worked alongside Mamello, Yandisa and the other women in my ethnography through TAC, as they called on the government to scale up the ARV roll-out. When Zukile started ARVs through the MSF trial in June 2001 he weighed 30 kilograms and his CD4 count was 174. He reflected the skeleton of his story in a body map that he created but did not complete in 2003. In 2011, he participated in an initiative to create a new body map. The 2011 body maps track the journey of each artist's life since starting ARVs and were placed in the waiting areas of Khayelitsha's hospital as mosaics; the artists' 2011 body maps bear witness to the legacy of their political and personal struggle to bring HIV medicines into the country's public health system, and into their own and their children's bodies.

In his 2011 body map, and in his speech at the MSF 10 Year Celebration, Zukile notes the change in his health over the last decade: in 2011, his CD4 count was 622 and his viral load was undetectable. These biomedical indicators connect to the life cycles of HIV and ARVs as actants, with ARVs having successfully prevented HIV from co-opting CD4 cells and replicating, thus supporting the CD4 cells in sustaining his immune system. In the contours of his body, he drew his source of strength: a spear, represented by a red sheath and a white handle. This spear, he said when describing the symbols in his map, represented his isiXhosa heritage and the way that he was encouraged (particularly through traditional male circumcision) to be strong. This is reflected in the message that he wrote for other people living with HIV: 'Life is a challenge – face it'. He attributes his emotional strength to his heritage and his physical strength to ARVs. The white markings in his body symbolise his ARVs. He said that he had been on ARVs for so long that they had become part of who he is; they were not simply pills that he put into his body – they *were* his body. ARVs had intra-acted so intimately with his body that he no longer distinguished between the boundaries of the medicine and the boundaries of his body – they had become each other.

His account draws into focus the biopolitical dynamic that linked the state of his body with the body of the state. As an activist, Zukile had called on the state to intervene in the space of his body by providing medicines; with these medicines, he had not only resumed full health but had also come to embody ARVs so fully that he no longer separated the boundaries of the pill from the state of his body. Lambert and McDonald (2009) consider, similarly, the shifts in attitudes towards the body that have followed technological developments, particularly those that have the capacity to 'remake life and death' (Franklin & Lock, 2003). Like Barad (2007), they challenge historical 'representationalist' approaches to embodiment in which the body is separated from the social and understood to be a slate for inscription. By foregrounding the entangled intra-action of HIV and ARVs with each other, illustrated in Zukile's body map and his account of ARVs, it becomes more possible to view the body as porous. His vitality is intimately entwined with a global assemblage that moved out his embodied experience of the intra-action of ARVs with the virus, to include a network of organisations (like MSF, TAC and Indian pharmaceutical companies) that spanned local, national and global levels.

Further, Zukile draws his cultural heritage, that of strength represented by a spear, within his body and alongside the ARVs that gave his body strength, disrupting dichotomies that separate the social from the science, discourse from materiality, human from non-human. Drawing on the definition of post-humanist performativity as 'one that incorporates important material and discursive, social and scientific, human and nonhuman, and natural and cultural factors' (Barad, 2003, p. 808), Zukile's account illustrates how – as non-human actant – ARVs moved into and become a part of his materiality, his body. The visual depiction of his body filled with ARVs illustrates the post-humanist dimension described by Barad (2003) as iterative intra-activity. Nowotny, Scott, and Gibbons (2001), too, reflect on the extent to which scientific knowledge becomes integrated into everyday life because, as Latour (2005) writes, science is 'internal' to rather than separate from society. Here, Zukile's body map similarly illustrates the extent to which scientific knowledge moves beyond an abstract set of concepts into the very space of his body and outwards, too, through his activism and leadership within TAC, and a speech he gave at the MSF ten year celebrations for example.

Andiswa, too, spoke of the impact of ARVs on her body and in her life through two body maps, one in 2003 and the second in 2011. I asked her about the white marks she had drawn in her 2011 body map. She said, 'These are the ARVs'. Tracing her hand over the red contour of her body, moving in and out of the white circles representing the ARVs, she echoed Zukile, saying, 'They're all over the body'. Andiswa's description suggests that the ARVs had, as with Zukile, become her body. By intra-acting with HIV, her ARVs were embodied in the fuller fleshier body she contrasts with her frail 'pre-ARV' self. As a way to describe how ARVs 'cooled' the fire of HIV, Andiswa echoed the other body map artists by referring to a set of biomedical indicators of relative illness and health that had changed between 2003 and 2011: 'My CD4 count was 18 at the time, and I was weighing 48 kg. This is me now, 2010, my CD4 count is 1045, my viral load is undetectable and I weigh 76 kilograms'. Andiswa's account, like Zukile's, suggests that the self-care practices entailed in adhering to ARVs were embodied by resumed health, indicated through these biomedical markers.

These markers suggest an 'internalisation' of scientific knowledge generated through TAC's treatment literacy programme: as ARVs prevent HIV from changing its genetic material and entering the CD4 cell, they enable healthy cells to support the body's immune response and quell the effect of HIV as a 'fire' that burns. MacGregor (2009) reflects on TAC's treatment literacy initiatives in light of this group's 2003 body maps and suggests that TAC's education activities reflect a 'context-sensitive' science. In the initial body maps, and now with this later set of maps, the narratives held in the women's body maps continue to reflect a sensitivity to the context in which people take ARVs; many of the women, for example, drew fruit and other foods on their maps and spoke about the importance of employment in supporting them to adhere to their treatment.

Across the body maps, ARVs were depicted as powerful non-human actants that had challenged the power of HIV within the arena of the body. Nokukhanya, for example, spoke about her sense of ARVs 'calming' the storm of HIV within her body through her body map in 2011:

> HIV is like nothing to me now. I'm not worried about it. Because I just see that it is calm. I show in this [2011] map that I'm walking up on – on top of – it. It's like the sand, you know, when you walk on the sand there is that mark... [With] wet sand it leaves a mark and then when the water comes it just wipes that mark. It's like the treatment that I already am taking has wiped the HIV. So now I don't feel like I have HIV. (Nokukhanya, 2011 fieldwork notes)

Nokukhanya's description of ARVs as radically transformative, an actant able to 'wipe HIV away', is a theme in many studies conducted just as ARVs became internationally available (Biehl, 2007, 2013; Rasmussen & Richey, 2012). Robins (2006), for example, refers to the 'treatment testimonies' of activists who give accounts of the 'lazarus effect' of HIV as they transitioned from bare life to full health. Their bare life was, Robins argues, a result of the state refusing to provide ARVs and therefore withholding their citizens' ability to secure long-term vitality; he links the 'lazarus effect', however, to both medicines and the responsibilities entailed in taking them. Similarly, although activists like Zukile, Andiswa and Nokukhanya accorded agency to ARVs, as actants, in their embodied health I found, too, that their resumed health was linked to a set of complex disciplining techniques in which the activity of ARVs with HIV within the body is played out, or performed.

These 'regimes of care' speak to Foucault's conception of 'technologies of the self' (Foucault, Martin, Gutman, & Hutton, 1988). He describes the 'techniques of self' prescribed by ancient Greek pagan morality in order to condition sexual ethics. His work has been taken up by anthropologists researching biomedical regimes of care to show a contradiction in the practices required of those receiving ARVs (Kalofonos, 2008). It has also been used by theorists in the field of critical public health to illuminate the frequently hidden, or taken for granted practices, of health practitioners to 'discipline' patients (Boyd & Kerr, 2015; Siconolfi, Halkitis, & Moeller, 2015). At the time of my fieldwork in South Africa, people on ARVs were told to follow a set of practices, a regime, that entailed strict adherence to their medicines and healthy eating. Unlike the Ancient Greeks, Marsland (2012) describes the contradiction she observed in Tanzania as those people with whom she worked were not moving from a place of decadence and plenty into one of ascetic restrictions; instead, they were required by biomedical regimes of care to – almost impossibly – secure scarce food and other material resources as techniques of 'positive living' on ARVs.

The people with whom I worked may have reflected Robins' (2006) description of compliant and 'responsibilised' citizen activists who, when starting ARVs a decade ago, committed to following a set of practices entailed in joining the MSF pilot trial. However, a decade later, we see that these practices of self-care are fraught and not simply a matter of 'compliance' or 'resistance' to biomedical regimes of care among the people with whom I worked. Through her research in Uganda, also with people receiving ARVs, Whyte (2009) similarly calls us to pay attention to the different contexts in which social, economic and biomedical subjectivities unfold.

Below, I turn to look into the body to see how, as actants, HIV and ARVs intra-act in complex ways with each other to generate risk and also opportunity. As we see in the following section, a new set of struggles have surfaced that problematise both the context in which ARVs intra-act with HIV 'within' the body, and the context in which people live that, too, is precariously embodied.

New generation struggles and embodied precarity

A number of the activists I hung out with referred to a prominent TAC activist who had become 'tired' and who had 'given up' taking his medication; it was a shock to them because he was well informed, worked to raise awareness around the efficacy of ARVs, and yet had reached a point where he was too 'tired' to continue taking his treatment. His treatment fatigue was also compounded by depression and alcoholism: he became very seriously ill with meningitis and asked to be placed back on ARVs, but by this stage his body had developed resistance to both lines of treatment and he died.

Treatment fatigue and viral resistance are two inter-linked 'new generation struggles' that emerged in my fieldwork. Participants frequently used the term 'tired' to describe their frustration with taking medicine at the same time, every day. Brenda, for example, decided to 'take a break' because she was tired of taking ARVs. During a conversation about the current government and changes in the politics of health, she said,

> If [President] Zuma could try to get third line I think it's good for us, or an injection. Because tablets are not easy to take. It's not easy to take ARV tablets every morning. That's why they have a lot of defaulters. So I think Zuma must try again or try harder to get something to help us. Because ARVs, wow! They're good, but if you take tablets... Yoh! You feel tired! (Brenda, 2011 fieldwork notes)

Brenda later found out that, as a result of interrupting her treatment, the virus had mutated sufficiently to outwit her first line ARVs and she was placed on second line treatment.

The artists of each of the body maps represented HIV in different ways inside their bodies. Andiswa, for example, drew HIV as the embers of a former conflagration, saying that ARVs had 'cooled' the fire down. Nokukhanya described HIV as the soft indentations of footprints on the wet sand, saying that ARVs had 'calmed' the storm of HIV down.

In contrast with all of the body maps developed in both 2003 and 2011, Nceba drew HIV outside her body. She said that now HIV was not what defined her and that, instead, it was a source of opportunity for her. HIV was symbolised by white ribbons around her body. Inside the ribbons she had drawn maple leaves; the leaves referred to the artistic collaborations that she had entered into with colleagues in Canada through her HIV activism and art. Her body map extends Zukile's description of ARVs as his body. Nceba, in an interview about her body map, said that ARVs had been so powerful that they had moved HIV outside her body. She pointed to the marks on her body, shown in the map as light brown markings along her legs and arms, saying, 'Yes, the effect of HIV is still on my skin, but HIV is not who I am'.

This marks a key shift in socialities as Nceba both claimed HIV through the kinds of opportunities she was able to access, while also asserting that she did not want to be fundamentally labelled as 'HIV-positive'. This further reflects Whyte's (2009) call to understand how subjectivities shift as people's embodied experience of illness changes. In Nceba's case, her experience of illness changed markedly after she accessed ARVs in 2002. In 2012, I visited Nceba, Andiswa and Zukile at an exhibition in London. They had worked with the British Council, in conjunction with the Paralympics, to develop a body of work with a British artist, Rachel Gadsen. We watched a performance, as part of this exhibition, where HIV took the form a dancer's body as she flew around the stage, wild and dangerous, before ARVs – another dancer – came to tame her.

As we see in Andiswa and Zukile's accounts, it is through the intra-action of ARVs with HIV that Nceba was able see HIV as 'beyond' her body. It is also, as I discuss above, through her discipline and self-care practices, particularly around adherence, that she was able to 'tame' HIV to the extent that she could 'see' it outside herself in the opportunities she was able to access. This presents another layer to the discussion above around Zukile's body map and post-humanist performativity as ARVs intra-act with HIV: it is through taking ARVs, every day, that Nceba 'saw' the presence of HIV in the form of her ARVs even as it was felt to be absent from her body.

This tension was a strong finding in my ethnography. In contrast with the notion of 'bare life' described by Robins (2006) and generated through the state's historical failure to provide essential ARVs, the way in which precarity was strategically performed by the research participants points to a different narrative. In connection with findings presented elsewhere on pathways of precarity where I suggest that instead of being either reduced to bare life or 'acted on' by national and international development programmes, women 'acted up' by strategically placing themselves within the 'development subjectivities' that had been discursively narrated through interventions and policies that framed women as economically, socially and biologically 'vulnerable' to HIV-infection (Mills, 2016).

When what is held in the body becomes social

The 10-year celebration of MSF's first ARV trial in Khayelitsha, in 2011, was a poignant and powerful marker of South Africa's shifting biopolitical landscape: at the time of my fieldwork, ARVs were no longer the scarce resource they were when people like Lilian, Zukile, Andiswa and Nceba first started taking these medicines a decade previously. It is for this reason, I propose, that we start to see a shift in the embodied accounts of the intra-action of HIV and ARVs in people's lives. This article traced these fluid accounts across time, and in relation to the people with whom I worked most closely during my fieldwork. It is therefore with the understanding that I worked with a particular group of people who were on ARVs and had engaged as activists in the historic context of the struggle for ARVs in South Africa, that I situate the following observations.

The article outlined how HIV and ARVs, as actants, were felt to within the body, and it illustrated how these actants are brought into the body through socialities that take place between multiple actors outside the body: in relationships between the people I worked with, TAC, MSF and the government. The socialities that were formed among the people with whom I worked around their HIV status was a strong feature of my fieldwork as I observed and took part in the networks of connection that brought friends and colleagues together.

Marsland (2012), Prince (2012), Meinert et al. (2009) and Le Marcis (2012), who have also researched ARV programmes in eastern and southern Africa in the decade following the initial struggle for ARVs, have suggested a reframing of the historical approach to biopolitics and biosociality. These medical anthropologists probe the limits of biopolitics as a 'one size fits all' conceptual approach, and suggest that 'biosocialities' are emergent, plural and should be understood in relation to the socio-economic contexts in which HIV-positive navigate their lives. In my own ethnography, context mattered. But I take context to matter both within and beyond the body, as I read the body itself as permeable.

Where my research connects to, but also moves from, even earlier accounts of HIV and biosociality is that, as actants, the post-humanist performativity of ARVs is not solely embodied in positive terms (described by Nguyen (2007, 2010) and Robins (2006)). Nor do these accounts highlight the limitations of biomedical programmes in places where people can sometimes simply not afford to take medicines that make them even more hungry and even less able to work (described by Marsland & Prince, 2012, for example). Thinking about ARVs as actants, things with a social life, highlights another form of sociality as they become felt by the people I worked with, and visible to other people, through their manifestation in side effects, like lipodystrophy. What is held in the body becomes social.

In conceptualising HIV and ARVs as actants, this article draws the social dimension of these actants lives into relief; further, 'new generation' struggles linked to adherence, viral resistance, side effects and socio-economic inequality bring the biological dimension of social, political and economic relationships into focus. For HIV not only enters women's lives through human relationships, but as an actant, HIV itself becomes alive and has, in Appadurai's (1988) terms, a 'social life' in the body. Once in the body, the virus learns to intra-act with the body's immune system and, over time, manages to con CD4 cells into mimicking the body's basic biological identity – its DNA. ARVs, like HIV, also call attention to the social, economic and political relationships that people navigated as activists in order to mobilise the government to bring these medicines into South Africa's public health system. However, once in the body, ARVs also took on a social life. They interacted with each other as they were technologically honed – as a triple therapy – to block HIV in its attempts to con the CD4 cells.

These actants intra-act and move into the social space of people's relationships with each other as they become visible as facets of sociality: through activist networks that mobilise around ARVs; around ARVs as they become embodied in people's physiological health and parallel side-effects; through the kind of sexual relationships that women can and cannot negotiate with their partners; through the economic resources they are able to secure by foregrounding one particular subjectivity – HIV – over the multitude of others; and through the emerging citizen claims that draw these women back into a biopolitical relationship with the state to access newer medical technologies that will have fewer negative effects on their bodies and that will be better able to combat HIV as it learns to outwit the older generation medicines. Therefore, the term 'diffracted biosocialities', rather than simply 'biosocialities', most accurately describes a dynamic connection across these facets (biological and social) and it denotes the complex ways in which the social is not only forged through biology, but where biology, itself, is social and forged through sociality.

In addition to the embodied precarity linked to side effects, viral resistance and adherence, the new generation struggles discussed in this article also relate to the socio-economic contours of these women's everyday lives. We see, in this strand of the new generation struggles, how HIV can and has been used performatively to secure, albeit precariously, resources through which women have been able to navigate the tightly stretched economic landscape in which they live.

Therefore, using ANT and post-humanist performativity as tools to explore the embodiment of biopolitical precarity, the paper reveals two overarching findings that, together, point to the value of moving away from the 'problem/solution' framing of HIV and ARVs (Lock & Nguyen, 2010). First, the findings suggest that although HIV can be a form of embodied precarity, it can also be a resource. Second, HIV – as an actant within the body – can also be performatively mobilised 'outside' through socio-economic relationships to manage precarity. In this regard, the women I worked with were able to strategically secure critical economic resources in a development milieu that perpetuates the 'gender/HIV' dyad (Mills, 2016). The article's findings suggest, then, that as 'local biologies' both HIV and ARVs have not only influenced the kind of social relationships that people form, but they too intra-act and perform social lives that are differentially embodied in people's lives.

Disclosure statement

No potential conflict of interest was reported by the author.

Funding

This work was supported by the Commonwealth Scholarship Commission.

References

Appadurai, A. (Ed.). (1988). *The social life of things: Commodities in cultural perspective*. Cambridge: Cambridge University Press.

Arendt, H. (1958). *The human condition*. Chicago, IL: University of Chicago.

Barad, K. (2003). Posthumanist performativity: Toward an understanding of how matter comes to matter. *Signs, 28*, 801–831.

Barad, K. (2007). *Meeting the universe halfway: Quantum physics and the entanglement of matter and meaning*. Durham, NC: Duke University Press Books.

Biehl, J. G. (2004). The activist state: Global pharmaceuticals, AIDS, and citizenship in Brazil. *Social Text, 22*, 105–132.

Biehl, J. G. (2007). *Will to live: AIDS therapies and the politics of survival*. Princeton, NJ: Princeton University Press.

Biehl, J. (2013). *Vita: Life in a zone of social abandonment*. Berkeley, CA: University of California Press.

Boyd, J., & Kerr, T. (2015). Policing 'Vancouver's mental health crisis': A critical discourse analysis. *Critical Public Health, 26*, 1–16.

Braidotti, R. (2013). *The posthuman*. Cambridge: Wiley.

Braidotti, R. (2016). Posthuman, all too human towards a new process ontology. *Theory, Culture & Society, 23*, 197–208.

Butler, J. (2004). *Undoing gender*. New York, NY: Routledge.

Butler, J. (2009). Performativity, precarity and sexual politics. *Antropólogos Iberoamericanos en Red (AIBR), 4*, i–xiii.

Collier, S. (2009). Topologies of power: Foucault's analysis of political government beyond 'governmentality'. *Theory, Culture & Society, 26*, 78–108.

Collier, S. J., & Ong, A. (2005). Global assemblages, anthropological problems. In A. Ong & S. J. Collier (Eds.), *Global assemblages: Technology, politics, and ethics as anthropological problems* (pp. 3–21). Oxford: Wiley-Blackwell.

Foucault, M. (1978). *The history of sexuality* (Vol. 1). New York, NY: Pantheon.

Foucault, M., Martin, L., Gutman, H., & Hutton, P. (1988). *Technologies of the self: A seminar with Michel Foucault*. Amherst, MA: University of Massachusetts Press.

Franklin, S., & Lock, M. (2003). *Remaking life & death: Toward an anthropology of the biosciences*. Oxford: John Currey.

Gilbert, H. (2013). Re-visioning local biologies: HIV-2 and the pattern of differential valuation in biomedical research. *Medical Anthropology, 32*, 343–358.

Gregson, N., & Rose, G. (2000). Taking Butler elsewhere: Performativities, spatialities and subjectivities. *Environment and Planning D, 18*, 433–452.

Hacking, I. (1990). *The taming of chance – Ideas in context*. Cambridge: Cambridge University Press.

Haraway, D. (1997). *Modest_Witness@Second_Millennium: FemaleMan_Meets_Oncomouse: Feminism and Technoscience*. New York, NY: Routledge.

Kalofonos, A. (2008). *"All I eat is ARVs": Living with HIV/AIDS at the dawn of the treatment era in Central Mozambique*. Ann Arbor, MI: ProQuest.

Lambert, H., & McDonald, M. (2009). *Social bodies*. New York, NY: Berghahn Books.

Latour, B. (2005). *Reassembling the social: An introduction to actor-network-theory*. Oxford: Oxford University Press.

Le Marcis, F. (2012). Struggling with AIDS in South Africa: The space of the everyday as a field of recognition. *Medical Anthropology Quarterly, 26*, 486–502.

Lock, M., & Nguyen, V.-K. (2010). *An anthropology of biomedicine*. Oxford: Wiley-Blackwell.

Loon, J. V. (2005). Epidemic space. *Critical Public Health, 15*, 39–52.

MacGregor, H. (2009). Mapping the body: Tracing the personal and the political dimensions of HIV/AIDS in Khayelitsha, South Africa. *Anthropology and Medicine, 16*, 85–95.

Marcus, G., & Saka, E. (2006). Assemblage. *Theory, Culture & Society, 23*, 101–106.

Marsland, R. (2012). (Bio)Sociality and HIV in Tanzania: Finding a living to support a life. *Medical Anthropology Quarterly, 26*, 470–485.

Marsland, R., & Prince, R. (2012). What is life worth? Exploring biomedical interventions, survival, and the politics of life. *Medical Anthropology Quarterly, 26*, 453–469.

Meinert, L., Mogensen, H. O., & Twebaze, J. (2009). Tests for life chances: CD4 miracles and obstacles in Uganda. *Anthropology and Medicine, 16*, 195–209.

Michael, M., & Rosengarten, M. (2012). HIV, globalization and topology: Of prepositions and propositions. *Theory, Culture & Society, 29*, 93–115.

Mills, E. (2016). When the skies fight: HIV, violence and pathways of precarity in South Africa. *Reproductive Health Matters, 24*, 85–95.

Nguyen, V.-K. (2007). Antiretroviral globalism, biopolitics, and therapeutic citizenship. In A. Ong & S. J. Collier (Eds.), *Global assemblages: Technology, politics, and ethics as anthropological problems* (pp. 124–144). Oxford: Blackwell.

Nguyen, V. K. (2010). *The republic of therapy: Triage and sovereignty in West Africa's time of AIDS*. Durham, NC: Duke University Press.

Nowotny, H., Scott, P., & Gibbons, M. (2001). *Re-thinking science: Knowledge and the public in an age of uncertainty*. Cambridge: Polity Press.

Prince, R. (2012). HIV and the moral economy of survival in an East African city. *Medical Anthropology Quarterly, 26*, 534–556.

Rasmussen, L. M., & Richey, L. A. (2012). The Lazarus Effect of AIDS treatment: Lessons learned and lives saved. *Journal of Progressive Human Services, 23*, 187–207.

Robins, S. (2005). AIDS, science and citizenship after apartheid. In M. Leach, I. Scoones, & B. Wynne (Eds.), *Science and citizens. Globalisation and the challenge of engagements* (pp. 113–115). London: Zed Books.

Robins, S. (2006). From "rights" to "ritual": AIDS activism in South Africa. *American Anthropologist, 108*, 312–323.

Robins, S. (2010). *From revolution to rights in South Africa: Social movements, NGOs & popular politics after apartheid*. Pietermaritzburg: Boydell & Brewer.

Siconolfi, D., Halkitis, P., & Moeller, R. (2015). Homo economicus: Young gay and bisexual men and the new public health. *Critical Public Health, 25*, 554–568.

Weber, M. (1984). *Legitimacy, politics and the state*. New York, NY: New York University Press.

Whyte, S. R. (2009). Health identities and subjectivities. *Medical Anthropology Quarterly, 23*, 6–15.

Beyond the person: the construction and transformation of blood as a resource

Rebecca Lynch and Simon Cohn

ABSTRACT

Many studies of blood donation have looked at the motives of donors, their relationship with the wider society and corresponding values such as gift-giving, altruism and responsibility. These underpin a rhetorical representation of person-to-person donation that neglects the many technical processes that take place between donation and eventual use and the material nature of blood itself. This ethnographic study, conducted in four UK blood donation sites, describes the various practices involved in routine sessions, rather than the motives or values or donors or staff. It focuses on the procedures and equipment that not only ensures blood is collected safely and efficiently, but the extent to which they determine the nature of the collected blood itself. Taking our cue from posthuman approaches, we argue donated blood as something that is 'made' only when it leaves the body; in other words, it is not simply extracted, but is constructed through specific practices. We illustrate how, as blood is separated from the body, it is increasingly depersonalised and reconstituted in order to have biomedical value. In this way, rather than reproducing the essentialist claim that blood is what social scientists often described as a 'special kind of substance', we point to the ways in which donated blood alters as it moves in time and space. We argue that such transformations occur in both symbolic and material realms, such that the capacity of blood to have both cultural meaning and clinical value is dependent on the fact that it is never stable or singular.

The seminal work by Titmuss on blood donation in the 1960s framed UK blood donation as voluntary and altruistic, in which donor and recipient are not known to each other (1970/1987). His argument is that this both reflects, and reproduces a sense of civic duty and fosters generalised social cohesion and continuity. However, rather than merely provide a sociological commentary, these sentiments have themselves become engrained in the ethos of the nation's blood service. The alignment between public health, blood as a public good and the ethics of civil society continue to be a key idiom adopted by participants in their motivation for donation (Busby, 2004; Cohn, 2016), and utilised by NHSBT (National Health Service Blood and Transplant, the UK national blood service) to promote, recruit and retain donors, often through their slogan of 'vein-to-vein' donation.

Whilst most people may well be aware that in practice blood is not transferred directly in this way, it remains a compelling representation that does a great deal of work. The motif of human-to-human donation is therefore a useful fiction, reinforced in posters, advertising and web pages. What is intriguing is that this narrative also continues to be reproduced in much of the social science research on the topic, which invariably focuses on the different ways the exchange of blood establishes social ties though its status as a gift (Healy, 2000; Mahon-Daly, 2012; Tran, Charbonneau, & Valderrama-Benitez, 2013; Wynne Busby, 2010). Over 30 years ago, Gregory (1982) noted that gift-based economies comprise exchanging 'inalienable' goods (objects that are invested with personhood and social relationships). In contrast, in order for objects to be bought and sold, they must not embedded in, or restricted by, social ties; hence, commodity-based economies exchange 'alienable' goods (objects without personal attachment). This perspective was taken up by Strathern, in her reflections on the social relations formed through the exchange of various bodily materials (1991). She proposed that while certain human tissues are inalienable, others circulate much like commodities because they are largely regarded as entities independent of persons; for example, in contrast to human eggs, she claims human kidneys are not thought about in terms of their social identity. Copeman, however, disagrees (2005), arguing that all human tissue and organs are inalienable to some degree, even if this manifests in different ways. According to him, although such things as donated kidneys or blood might appear to circulate as impersonal objects, the very powerful motives and meanings donors invest in their acts of donation cannot be neglected, even if they are not always carried overtly along with the donated material (2005, p. 479).

Between these opposing stances, Waldby suggests that human tissues such as donated stem cells and blood are never either commodities or gifts (2002), pointing out not only that these different spheres of exchange usually co-exist, but that there is rarely a clear demarcation between them. She suggests that what should be attended to instead is the circulation of new forms of 'biovalue' which are rapidly emerging from the 'biotechnical reformulation of living processes'. Nevertheless, in common with all these positions, the issues of anonymity and personhood are presented as key to determining the alienability or otherwise of substances such as blood, and therefore the manner in which it might circulate. And in keeping with Gregory's original concern, it is assumed that the determination of this is a cultural process, irrespective of its material nature.

In contrast to this, our argument is that matters of alienability are not solely determined by a substance's symbolic value, and that producing blood for future clinical use or research requires a combination of material as well as semiotic transformations. If one fails to consider the extent to which blood materially alters as it is collected and redistributed, the same fiction that donors and the blood service draw on is inadvertently reproduced. Berner (2010) provides a fascinating historical account of developments of blood transfusion over the first half of the twentieth century, during which time the increasing number of medical techniques and interventions embedded the donor and recipient in more and more complex sociotechnical assemblages. The result was that the donor became increasingly separated from the recipient, both physically and temporally. Our paper complements this insight, but focuses on the contemporary ways in which routine procedures not only separate donors' blood from their body, but how this separation in inescapably coupled with its material alteration. In this way, it problematises any description that final blood products simply come from a donor's body.

This approach draws on shifts over recent years from a diverse range of perspectives to reframe conventional social sciences approaches by not assuming the human is necessarily the principle agent in social and cultural events (e.g. Braidotti, 2015; Wolfe, 2010). Such approaches have included thinking about the role of non-human organisms, and the relationships they have with humans (Haraway, 2008); the significance of material objects and the extent to which their physical properties shape how events unfold (Barad, 2007); and more generally, how any specific context is not merely the background for a discrete set of agents, but is a heterogeneous field which actively determines the formation and configuration of agents themselves (Puig de la Bellacasa, 2011). Arguably one of the most famous essays which set out much of this intellectual agenda was by Callon in his discussion of French fisherman, scallops, and attempts to farm them (Callon, 1984). In this account, he describes the ways in which different elements – humans, objects, physical environments and non-human organisms – relate and associate with each other in such intricate ways that often human agency and even political potential are dependent on the manner in which many non-human elements may 'choose' to act. A key point he raises is that in the making of relationships, the 'identity and characteristics of the implicated actors change as well'.

Overall, this broad literature, which has collectively been described as 'posthuman', does not dismiss human accounts, but rather recognises the productive value of resisting traditional assumptions about what is significant, valuable, or relevant. Our view, therefore, is that the term itself can often be unhelpful, in that it suggests a primary interest in people is unequivocally displaced by these new orientations: This is not necessarily the case. What is more crucial is that such approaches remain vigilant to the many nonhuman elements – for example, the physical environment and role of material objects – since they do not simply enable human action, but form an integral part of what that action is and can do. Following Latour (2005), this produces a radically different notion of what should constitute social enquiry because it emphasises the heterogeneity of potential actors and members of the social, inviting a fuller, and indeed more inclusive, ethnography (Panelli, 2010). As Mol has pointed out, social researchers often forget about the many other actors in the room (Mol, 2002). By broadening the scope of enquiry not only to include non-human elements but recognise them as potential actors, humans may be said to be decentred. But this does not mean that our primary matter of concern, rather than scope of enquiry, can no longer continue to be that relating to humans and their health.

The value of adopting this perspective to think about blood donation is not only that we might resist falling into the trap of thinking of donation in terms of the simple exchange from one person to another. It might also engage with the significant modernisation of services in recent years within the UK and internationally, that has led to the introduction of new equipment, new practices and ultimately new forms of biovalue (Alliance of Blood Operators, n.d.; Australian Red Cross Blood Service, 2014). Changes to biomedical science and research are shifting the relations between the commercial sector, public health care and the individual; as a result, discourses of waste and efficiency are increasingly being combined with those of gift-giving and altruism (Tupasala, 2011). Developments are also influencing the demand for blood, and in particular the traffic of specific blood components and products in a global 'technoscape' (Appadurai, 1996). At a national level, while the UK blood service is typically associated with small mobile donation sites in local communities, it is progressively placing greater emphasis on electronical appointment sessions run from custom-built static centres, which are better able to respond to fluctuations in demand for blood and blood products. Coupled to this, increased attention is being paid to the 'safe donation experience', promoting a 'modern, attractive and easy to use service', ensuring 'high levels of customer service' and 'reducing the variation in experience for donors' (NHSBT a, n.d.). NHSBT working papers use phrases such as developing a 'lean national supply chain' and 'minimising wastage, reduce infrastructure costs and minimise non-productive time' (NHSBT b, n.d.). Accordingly, new protocols, equipment and procedures are being introduced to ensure donation sessions are as efficient as possible and increasingly able to respond to contemporary demands.

However, rather than address these developments through an argument of globalising 'neoliberal' processes of efficiency and homogenisation (Bell & Green, 2016; Will, 2017), we instead examine the effects that these forces shape local practice, and the way relatively small technical procedures serve to enact them. Against the backdrop of a complex and distributed international system of blood exchange, there may well be increasing dissonance with the traditional vein-to-vein, human-to-human, motif, demanding new ways to think about blood, its movement and its value. As a consequence, we are interested in the ways that these changes may relate to, or clash with, the continued promotion of social and cultural meanings attached to blood and blood donation. This paper therefore asks to what extent might the growing imperative to increase the biovalue of blood in the national and international market, as articulated by ideas of efficiency and leanness, inevitably strip the social and cultural values from donated blood.

Methodology

In this paper, we draw on ethnographic observations of donation sessions and interviews with donors. This approach allows examination not only of what people say and do, but also the active role materials, objects and technologies have. Donation sessions in four of NHSBT's current 24 static centres established were observed over eight months; one based in a community hospital, two in large hospital sites (one urban, one more rural) and the fourth within an urban shopping centre. The purpose was not to compare these sites, but rather identify those aspects of procedure, equipment and practice that they had in common. Our approach was inspired by the much-cited advice from Actor Network Theory to 'follow the actor' (Latour, 2005) – in our case, the flow of blood. However, knowing that there were many different, if apparently minor, procedures and practices involved in determining who might donate and what blood was acceptable, our approach was not simply to record what networks blood became enmeshed in, but rather how those interactions served to constitute blood in particular ways. In other words, by taking blood to be our ethnographic focus, rather than the people, our analysis attended to changes in matter, and well as meaning.

We also observed various NHSBT meetings, chatted informally to staff (donor carers, nurses, centre managers and receptionists) and conducted interviews with 30 regular blood donors about their experiences. The donors were drawn from participants in a randomised control trial looking at the impact of increased frequency of donations on blood supply and donor health (the INTERVAL trial; for more information see Moore et al., 2014) and were purposefully sampled to reflect a range of ages and balance of gender. The in-depth semi-structured interviews were conducted by RL, lasted between 45 and 145 min and were audio-recorded prior to thematic coding and analysis. Verbatim transcriptions were imported into NVivo 10 alongside the field notes. All data were initially coded using themes from the interview guide and then using more analytical codes which emerged through systematically reading and rereading the transcripts. RL and SC discussed and refined these iteratively in order to establish higher level themes. Throughout the study we were sensitive to the needs and positioning of donors and donation centre staff, ensuring that we did not impede their activities, and only directly observed or interviewed individuals after explicit consent to do so. Formal NHS ethical approval was obtained for this study.

Below, we bring together the observations, reflections from the interviews, and descriptions of some of the techniques, protocols and materials involved in contemporary blood donation to give an account that centres on the non-human elements of donation, and the ways in which these interact with human actors to produce certain material entities. In so doing, we detail how blood undergoes a series of necessary alterations in order that it will be suitable for recipients at a later date. The process begins with separating bodies from persons, then blood from bodies, and finally a separation of blood itself. These processes of separation and division are also accompanied by various additions and modifications. We consequently highlight how blood is never a singular or essential substance, but is always a composite that can always be further divided or augmented to produce new biomedical potential.

Separating bodies from people

Individual donation sessions follow a national standardised procedure developed by NHSBT that stipulates not only the order of various steps, but many other details, such as the arrangement of equipment and layout of furniture. Instructions are designed to make the process as seamless and orchestrated as possible. In doing so, the clear linear ordering not only plots out the various stages and techniques, but communicates the overall message that successful sessions are about managing throughput and the efficient attainment of blood.

Potential donors must be aged between 17 and 66 if it's their first time, although currently there is no upper age limit for existing donors. Before any physical tests are conducted, they must all complete a preliminary form called the 'Donor Health Check'. This requires them to tick boxes about their lifestyle, sexual behaviour, current health status, medication, and periods of travel outside the UK. Everyone is aware that the questionnaire is designed to screen out people who might have a high risk of blood-borne infection: those who have had recent piercings or tattoos; who have travelled to particular countries where the likelihood of contracting certain illnesses are higher; those who have injected drugs; or might be at risk of carrying HIV because of their recent sexual activity. In this way, completing the form already starts to select those who can donate from those who cannot. But throughout much of the promotional work it does, the blood service is very careful about navigating between, on the one hand, being able to reassure people it is continually vigilant about the safety of its procedures and products, and on the other animating people's sense of good will and altruistic intentions. It is an almost impossible tension; some people object to filling in the questionnaire or to certain specific questions, while others may see the need in general, but take offence that somehow they themselves are not being trusted.

A brief private follow-up interview by a qualified nurse goes over the responses to confirm suitability. Those deemed to be 'low risk' then have a droplet of blood taken to test whether they have sufficient levels of haemoglobin. A finger is pricked and a blood droplet dripped into a blue-coloured aqueous copper sulphate solution. Its specific gravity means that only blood containing a sufficient amount iron is able to descend. If the blood fails to sink, a follow-up test is done using blood from a vein and an electronic meter. Anyone confirmed to have low levels of iron, and who might potentially be diagnosed anaemic, is told to come back after some weeks. Again, NHSBT is very conscious of the potential effects of deferring people in this way, and the fact that some people may experience this as rejection so never return. So when this does occur, nurses generally follow a scripted response to encourage the potential donor to come back, reflecting the fact that retaining an active donor population is a constant problem, as newly recruited donors tend to be continually offset by those who no longer turn up.

Through these initial routine stages of selection there is a clear progression from engaging with the donor as a person, by asking questions about their lifestyle and behaviour, to increasingly concentrating on the body and the nature of the blood it contains. In this way, persons are progressively separated from their bodies. The various arrangements and items of kit are key to a process designed to protect the safety of donors and guard against any possible contamination of the blood; from the question-naire, to the iron test, the focus of attention shifts from care about the lifestyle and experiences of the donors to care of the body as a container of blood. The staff, too, are part of this selection technology. However, they find the task of selecting donors from those who have made the effort to come, but have to be turned away, tricky. Matters relating to the cultural and the biological have to be divided, as the symbolic significance of blood drawn on to encourage people to come potentially conflicts with having to assess bodies and blood according to different criteria.

Those judged as being able to donate have to wait until a slot becomes available. They are then greeted by a donor carer, and walked over to a specially designed chair. The chairs are increasingly being used at centres because they have been specifically designed to provide a safer and more ergo-nomic alternative to the traditional beds, which offered limited adjustment and couldn't always prevent donors from falling off. The chair can be swung rearward to help prevent fainting, or reclined fully to allow recovery should this occur (fainting occurs in around 300 blood donors in a typical donation day, SEE Platform [Sharing Experience Europe], 2014). Once seated, the carer checks the details on donor's form, and makes sure that everything matches on the multiple sets of labels that will be used. A sealed collection set is then opened. Described as a 'Whole Blood Collection and Component Storage System', it is made up of a main blood bag (which contains an anticoagulant and an additive to ensure the blood remains viable), a sample pouch, tubing and a catheter needle. The contents are carefully inspected, checked to see it is in date, and that there is no sign of moisture (which may indicate a leak).

Then, during the actual period of taking blood, donors freely allow their allotted carers to take control, touching and moving their bodies to determine how things should proceed. The carer normally asks which arm the donor would like the blood to be taken from. A conversation about veins might then ensue while a tourniquet is put on, pulled taut, and a suitable vein is felt for. Frequently, the donor and staff member inspect the arm jointly; in so doing, the limb is presented between them as a common, but distinct, object. The language used also reflects this somewhat detached assessment, with regular comments about which veins might be 'good' or 'problematic' depending on whether they are thought able to hold the standard-sized needle and facilitate a good flow. Some donors even boast about the speed at which their arm or blood vessels can usually fill a blood bag (usually between 5 and 10 min). In this way, through the joint interaction between the donor and staff, it is now the physical proper-ties of the person's body which are now being scrutinised. While the cuff maintains pressure, and the puncture site is checked for skin lesions and made sterile, a 16-gauge cannula needle is taken out of its tamper-proof cover. At this point, although some donors cast their gaze away, but many watch with fascination as it enters the arm and blood is drawn. First, a small amount flows through the collection tubing into a sample pouch. Being physically part of the collection kit, this in-line system reduces overall donation time and any risk of bacterial contamination. But once a sample has been collected, a permanent clamp is clicked shut (which will allow for the pouch to be snapped off later) and the flow diverted to the main collection bag.

While a few may continue to avert their eyes as the blood flows, most are clearly intrigued, looking with interest as their blood streams down the tube into the blood bag. Some donors spoke afterwards about the uncanny feeling of blood flowing from their arm, and that its warmth though the tubing felt particularly strange against their cooler skin. As the blood is collected donors may watch televisions positioned above them, read, or use the internet on their phones. To ensure the blood, anticoagulant and additive are gently mixed together, the blood bag is retained in a rocking agitator that inverts it every 60 s. It makes a gentle repetitive mechanical noise. Staff who had worked in the service for a long time recalled how, before these devices were introduced, the mixing of blood and anticoagulant had to be done by hand continuously until the bag was full. Regulating this is now an automated process, as the agitator also constantly weighs the blood and then stops, emitting warning beeps, when 470–475 ml has been collected.

Despite this degree of standardisation, individual carer staff often have their own preferred ways of using the equipment; for example, differing slightly in the ways in which they may place the tape on an arm to hold the needle or 'tricks' to improve the standard venepuncture protocol by arranging the tubing in particular locations to aid flow. The brief chats with the donor, constant attention to the arm, and regular checking of the equipment, are ways in which staff move between caring for the donor, caring for the body, and caring for the blood as it is produced. It is their role to manage these distinct remits: to produce a full bag of blood filled to correct levels and mixed with coagulant; a body which produced a timely and continuous flow of blood without incident; and a person who doesn't feel unwell or faint.

Because identical equipment has to be used – the same needle for big or small veins, the same chairs for tall or short bodies, the same volume blood bag – their design mean that occasionally staff are unsuccessful in collecting a full bag of blood. Sometimes a suitable vein cannot be found, or the flow is too sluggish, or occasionally the donor feels such discomfort that the procedure has to be halted. This means that, in practice, staff consider donation to be generally easier from male donors (who typically have larger veins) and people who are not too small. When asked about this, one donor carer simply responded by saying 'you can't change the equipment, you have to change the body', referring to the fact that on rare occasions if they fail in collecting blood from someone they simply move on to the next person waiting. In this way, the design of the technology does not simply reflect norms but also operationalises them, itself sorting out variations of persons and bodies into those that are able to donate from those which cannot. In so doing, different elements interact – the chair, the arm, a cannula, a vein – each of which can contribute to determining not only how the blood will be collected, but the very nature of the collected blood itself.

Once the rocking agitator machine indicates that the bag is full, the carer deflates the pressure cuff, removes the catheter, tubing and blood bag from the arm, and asks the donors to hold a cotton swab over their puncture site. The needle is placed in a specialised disposal container and the blood bag is gently inverted a few more times by hand to make sure its contents have been thoroughly mixed. Donors are told briefly about how to look after their bodies; they are advised to keep pressure on the bandage, drink plenty of fluids, rest and not exert themselves, not drive immediately, and not have a hot bath that day. They are warned to look out for feeling light-headed or dizzy, in which case they should lie down immediately. And after this, they are directed towards a seating area to have a cup of tea or fruit drink and a biscuit to recover: time, liquid and sugar all designed to avoid the possibility of fainting.

While the donor rests, the carer takes the blood bag and sample pouch to the packaging area. Here it is categorised by type and Rhesus status, and the data added to charts and tallies in order to see how the session compares to the weekly targets set for different blood types. Already by this stage of the donation procedure, the blood has undergone processes and operations which not only separate it from the donor, but have changed its material nature and qualities. It is mixed with new substances and contained in different vessels that alter its physical characteristics; for example, as it cools it no longer coagulates because of new chemical bonds that have been introduced, and the cells do not die rapidly. And in this form it now has new biomedical potentials.

Separating blood itself

When talking about the donation process afterwards, donors convey little sense of ownership of their blood once it has left their arm, with only a few reflecting on whether they even saw a van or bike transporting blood away. The blood is packed into cool bags and picked up by specially trained couriers and taken to one of the large national processing centres, while the sample pouch is sent separately for testing at sites which provide high throughput laboratory analysers for signs of HIV, hepatitis B and C, Human T-cell Lymphotropic Virus (HTLV), and syphilis. The advanced IT system, called 'Pulse', ensures barcode linkage between this and the trajectory of the main donation – what is frequently termed 'traceability'. Although not a secret, NHSBT rarely talks about processing centres in its promotional materials. They are large, industrial-like buildings, housing staff and machinery, including long conveyor belts, crates of blood bags and robotic handling in large open spaces.

A key element of what NHSBT call the 'blood supply chain' is the main PVC bag itself. It has been designed not only for collecting the blood but also for transit and processing, thereby maintaining a 'closed system' to minimise waste or the possibility of contamination. The flexible bags are strong enough to ensure they do not accidentally tear or burst, yet are also permeable because platelets need oxygen to survive, and are heat resistant so they can sterilised using steam (a cheaper method than radiation sterilisation). This relatively simple technology has had a great effect on NHSBT operations, allowing for a high degree of automation throughout various stages, and making direct human intervention redundant. It enables blood processing to be conducted 24 h a day, seven days a week using advanced systems in blood filtration, conveyor and storage system.

At the processing centre, the bagged blood is sorted, registered, and then sent to what NHSBT terms 'the manufacturing area'. Small amounts of rare blood types may be frozen whole, but most blood is separated into different components. Having filtered out white cells, the bag is centrifuged or 'pressed' to divide – or 'fractionate' – red blood cells, plasma and platelets into different packs that are sealed and detached from each other. These different substances are then held in 'quarantine' until the results of the blood test confirms whether they can be used. After this, the packs are placed in storage, where an even temperature distribution is maintained and vibrations, which might damage the blood components, are minimised. The requirements of each vary, further illustrating the extent to which they are now discrete entities. Red blood cells can be kept for 42 days at a temperature of between 2 and 6 °C; the platelets only last up to seven days and are stored in incubators at room temperature and are agitated once a second to prevent clumping; and finally the yellowish plasma is frozen at below −18 °C, known as cryoprecipitate, where it remains viable for a year.

This description shows how the blood produced at local centres is now combined and divided in new ways as it is filtered, separated, and tested, to be radically transformed. NHSBT describe these technological manipulations as 'manufacture', creating substances that are more and more distinct from the blood that was once circulating in the donor. But it is only through these manipulations that the products have the potential to circulate in different bodies. Each will go on to be used for different purposes; the red blood cells are mostly used for trauma and surgery, but also for treating anaemia, blood loss and for blood disorders such as sickle cell anaemia; platelets are generally used for cancer treatments and organ transplants; while the plasma is commonly used to treat liver and kidney disease and bleeding disorders such as haemophilia. These products have not simply been 'extracted' *from* the blood; while they were in the blood bags they existed in combined form as donated blood. Now, they exist in their new forms through processes involving humans and nonhuman to enable them to materialise, be stored and transported in new ways.

Discussion

At the beginning of this paper, we outlined how overly human-centred accounts of blood donation give the impression that blood is inevitably a special substance and is afforded with an exceptional status because of its intrinsic cultural and symbolic positioning. NHSBT often reproduces this motif when promoting the service and seeking new donors by focusing on how a person giving blood can 'save a life' and establish a direct person-to-person tie with an anonymous recipient.[1] Our paper has been an attempt to address two aspects of that representation which has led to much research focusing solely on the cultural symbolism of blood donation and its social meaning. The first is that this concentrates on human actors at the expense of many other elements that are just as significant for blood to be successfully collected, distributed and used. And the second is that it depicts a continuity of the material nature of blood throughout the stages of exchange. In contrast, by attending to the mundane, material aspects of blood donation our ethnography describes some of those aspects frequently left out. We have drawn on a posthumanism sensibility to de-centre the role of the donor and highlight particular elements and relationships not normally included. In particular, we have described not only the various stages of material transformation, but the ways in which these have to be accomplished without completely undermining the social and cultural representations of blood donation.

As a feature of these processes, we illustrated how particular entities are divided and excluded – types of persons, types of bodies and types of blood – and how other entities come together – the vein and the cannula, blood and coagulant, white blood cells and a filter, etc. Through these interactions, new forms of blood are produced. The processes alter its composition, location, temperature and potential capacities. The point is that in accounts that describe the movement of blood from one location to another, and from one time point to another, it cannot be one, stable, substance; like all entities, as it travels it inevitably alters (see Williams, 2013). The stages of production, distribution and consumption, drawn on in many accounts of commodities, including pharmaceuticals and biological products, tend to present them in a simple linear fashion, leading to a focus on such things as medicalisation, pharmaceuticalisation, regulation and consumption (see for example, Williams, Gabe, & Davis, 2008). But thinking about donation as the first of these would keep particular actors and bodies separate, presenting blood as a stable substance that passes along from one to the next. In our study, many aspects of transportation, distribution and the future use of the blood determined by national and global forces shape the practices of donation itself.

The result is that blood is continuously manipulated as a range of actions alter and transform its capacities and potentials; it is stored and tested, has products added and components removed, is frozen, separated and reassembled, and is transported from arm to bag, and from local donation sites to national processing centres. Although blood may well continue to be a powerful signifier for such things as kinship, race and the social collective, and ideas of stability and continuity, its biovalue is entirely dependent on a continual chain of transformations. It is precisely this status of blood as a separated and technological set of products that means it can be used by others. The stripping away of some of its biological entanglements with the donor – through processes of selection, filtration, separation and mixing – enables it to then amalgamate with different human bodies at a later date. One reading of this might be to suggest that the transformations of blood produce substances that are themselves 'post' human and less 'natural' than the blood circulating in a donor's body. However, whilst these may initially appear to be processes that make the blood more 'pure' and uniform, less 'individual' and entirely alienable, we want to argue that instead what is happening is that different human dimensions are being introduced as others are foreclosed.

Although the practices of blood donation may well disentangle aspects of the individual donor from the blood, this is not a simple process of purification to produce blood in some kind of unadulterated state. The clinic and its documents, the specially designed chairs, the courier van with trained driver, the processing centre with its conveyor belts and centrifuges are all enfolded in the bloods they enact because they determine the nature of the substances that advance, and those that do not. It is not simply that the design of the equipment, the protocols of the donor carers, and even the automated systems of blood product manufacture are designed by humans, but that they fashion the materialisation of blood in particular ways. In this way, the transformed blood is no less human – it is just less of one particular human. This point shows how materialist accounts therefore go hand-in-hand with more human-centric accounts, rather than conflict with them. The very existence of blood in separated forms, in bags, kept at specific temperatures, and mixed with new substances, relies entirely on a wide range of technical human operations. Consequently, it makes little sense to oppose what is human from what is nonhuman, what is inalienable from what is alienable, since, paradoxically, one term does not simply define the other, but enables it. We therefore are not suggesting that the symbolic aspects of blood and blood donation – relating to such things as life, vitality, vigour and rescue – are simply mistaken because donated blood is not the substance it is assumed to be. Rather, our study points to the fact that essentialist accounts of blood are themselves predicated on the fluidity and multiplicity of the substance itself. In other words, cultural ideas of blood as being tied to personhood, and indeed more general accounts of being human as a singular and stable entity at all, can only be maintained in everyday life by virtue of the fact that material forms constantly reconfigure, adapt and alter.

At the beginning, we asked whether changes to the blood service, which increasingly are adopting the language of efficiency, production, and manufacture, might clash with existing cultural ideas associated with the donation of blood and saving the life of another person. Certainly, our account touched on occasions when either individual staff members or the organisation itself struggles to divide these two logics. But many of the biotechnical material manipulations and interventions that enable blood to be associated with ideas of social stability and continuity are already witnessed by donors and part of the imagery that NHSBT draw on. This suggests people do not experience these different spheres of meaning – the efficient manufacture of blood products and giving the gift of life – as necessarily contradictory. Rather, it may well be that values of human health are already seen to rely on other kinds of value, that intersect and enable what it means to be human, and what it means to be healthy. This closing observation is an important one for public health. To think beyond the human, by paying particular attention to other non-human actors, does not necessarily mean that public health is no longer primarily concerned with the health of people. But it does point to the fact that how we might value human health, and act to improve it, is always dependent on things we define as not being human. And, as we have shown, people are always embedded in the social, but the world of the social is not solely human.

Ethics

Ethical approval was granted by the National Research Ethics Service Committee East of England – Cambridge East (Research Ethics Committee (REC) reference 11/EE/0538).

Acknowledgements

The authors would like to thank all donors who kindly gave up their time to be interviewed as well as the managers and staff of the blood donation centres for their assistance and hospitality. A version of this paper was presented as part of a panel on post-human approaches in anthropology at the EASA/RAI medical anthropology conference in September 2015 and we are grateful for the comments of participants on this paper. In addition, the authors are grateful for the assistance and guidance of those involved in running the INTERVAL blood donation study, particularly Professor John Danesh, Carmel Moore, Zoe Tolkien and Rachel Henry at the University of Cambridge, and Gayle Miflin at NHSBT. Participants in the INTERVAL trial were recruited with the active collaboration of NHS Blood and Transplant (NHSBT) England (www.nhsbt.nhs.uk). Investigators at the University of Oxford have been supported by the Research and Development Programme of NHSBT, the NHSBT Howard Ostin Trust Fund, and NIHR Oxford Biomedical Research Centre.

Note

1. In Sweden, this has been reinforced through a campaign which sends donors a text when their blood has been used for another person. Here the processing and splitting that donated blood undergoes is not flagged up but rather the direct link between donor and recipient is maintained.

Disclosure statement

No potential conflict of interest was reported by the authors.

Funding

This work was funded as part of the INTERVAL blood donation trial. INTERVAL was supported by core funding from: NIHR Blood and Transplant Research Unit in Donor Health and Genomics, UK Medical Research Council [G0800270]; British Heart Foundation (SP/09/002); and NIHR Cambridge Biomedical Research Centre.

References

Alliance of Blood Operators. (n.d.). *2014–2019 strategic plan*. Retrieved August 23, 2016, from https://allianceofbloodoperators. org/media/101721/ABO-Strategic-Plan-2014-FINAL.pdf

Appadurai, A. (1996). *Modernity at large: Cultural dimensions of globalization*. Minneapolis: University of Minnesota Press.

Australian Red Cross Blood Service. (2014). *At the leading edge: Strategic plan 2014–2019*. Retrieved August 23, 2016, from http://www.donateblood.com.au/sites/default/files/Strategic_Plan_2014-2019_At_the_Leading_Edge.pdf

Barad, K. (2007). *Meeting the universe halfway: Quantum physics and the entanglement of matter and meaning*. Durham, NC: Duke University Press.

Bell, K., & Green, J. (2016). On the perils of invoking neoliberalism in public health critique. *Critical Public Health, 26*, 239–243.

Berner, B. (2010). (Dis) connecting bodies: Blood donation and technical change, Sweden 1915–1950. In E. Johnson & B. Berner (Eds.), *Technology and medical practice: Blood, guts and machines* (pp. 179–201). Farnham: Ashgate.

Braidotti, R. (2015). *The posthuman*. Cambridge: Polity Press.

Busby, H. (2004). Blood donation from genetic research: What can we learn from donors' narratives? In R. Tutton & O. Corrigan (Eds.), *Genetic databases: Socio-ethical issues in the collection and use of DNA* (pp. 39–56). London: Routledge.

Callon, M. (1984). Some elements of a sociology of translation: Domestication of the scallops and the fishermen of St Brieuc Bay. *The Sociological Review, 32*, 196–233.

Cohn, S. (2016). Blood and the public body: A study of UK blood donation and research participation. *Critical Public Health, 26*, 24–35.

Copeman, J. (2005). Veinglory: Exploring processes of blood transfer between persons. *Journal of the Royal Anthropological Institute, 11*, 465–485.

Gregory, C. A. (1982). *Gifts and commodities*. London: Academic Press.

Haraway, D. (2008). *When species meet*. Minneapolis: University of Minnesota Press.

Healy, K. (2000). Embedded altruism: Blood collection regimes and the European Union's donor population. *American Journal of Sociology, 105*, 1633–1657.

Latour, B. (2005). *Reassembling the social: An introduction to Actor-Network-Theory*. Oxford: Oxford University Press.

Mahon-Daly, P. M. (2012). *Blood, society and the gift* (A thesis submitted for the degree of Doctor of Philosophy by Patricia Mary Mahon-Daly). London: Brunel University.

Mol, A. (2002). *The body multiple: Ontology in medical practice*. Durham, NC: Duke University Press.

Moore, C., Sambrook, J., Walker, M., Tolkien, Z., Kaptoge, S., Allen, D., et al. (2014). The INTERVAL trial to determine whether intervals between blood donations can be safely and acceptably decreased to optimise blood supply: Study protocol for a randomised controlled trial. *Trials, 15*, 363.

NHSBT a. (n.d.). *Blood 2020. A strategy for the blood supply in England and North Wales*. Retrieved March 23, 2016, from http://www.nhsbt.nhs.uk/download/blood-2020.pdf

NHSBT b. (n.d.). *Strategic plan 2013–18*. Retrieved March 23, 2016, from http://www.nhsbt.nhs.uk/download/nhsbt-strategic-plan-201318.pdf

Panelli, R. (2010). More-than-human social geographies: Posthuman and other possibilities. *Progress in Human Geography, 34*, 79–87.

Puig de la Bellacasa, M. (2011). Matters of care in technoscience: Assembling neglecting things. *Social Studies of Science, 41*, 85–106.

SEE Platform [Sharing Experience Europe]. (2014). *Case study on blood donation*. Retrieved June 10, 2016, from http://www.seeplatform.eu/casestudies/Blood%20Donation%20Chair

Strathern, M. (1991). Partners and consumers: Making relations visible. *New Literary History, 22*, 581–601.

Strathern, M. (2009). Afterword (to special issue on blood). *Body and Society, 15*, 1–28.

Titmuss, R. (1987). *The gift relationship: From human blood to social policy*. London: George, Allen and Unwin.

Tran, N. Y. L., Charbonneau, J., & Valderrama-Benitez, V. (2013). Blood donation practices, motivations and beliefs in Montreal's Black communities: The modern gift under a new light. *Ethnicity & Health, 18*, 508–529.

Tupasala, A. (2011). From gift to waste: Changing policies in biobanking practices. *Science and Public Policy, 38*, 510–520.

Waldby, C. (2002). Stem cells, tissue cultures and the production of biovalue. *Health: An Interdisciplinary Journal for the Social Study of Health, Illness and Medicine, 6*, 305–323.

Will, C. M. (2017). On difference and doubt as tools for critical engagement with public health. *Critical Public Health, 27* (3).

Williams, J. (2013). *Gilles Deleuze's difference and repetition: A critical introduction and guide*. Edinburgh: Edinburgh University Press.

Williams, S. J., Gabe, J., & Davis, P. (2008). The sociology of pharmaceuticals: Progress and prospects. *Sociology of Health & Illness, 30*, 813–824.

Wolfe, C. (2010). *What is Posthumanism?* Minneapolis: University of Minnesota Press.

Wynne Busby, H. (2010). Trust, nostalgia and narrative accounts of blood banking in England in the 21st century. *Health, 14*, 369–382.

Technologies of the self in public health: insights from public deliberations on cognitive and behavioural enhancement

P. Lehoux, B. Williams-Jones, D. Grimard and S. Proulx

ABSTRACT

The aim of this paper is to examine how members of the public define the legitimacy of cognitive and behavioural enhancement. Our study involved a two-step multimedia-based deliberative intervention in which participants of different age groups pondered the desirability of a fictional enhancement technology: a sweater made of 'smart' textiles that provide 'bio-psycho-feedback' (PBF) to its user. A 3-min video clip presenting the fictional technology was used to stimulate deliberations in four face-to-face workshops ($n = 38$). A larger group of participants ($n = 57$) then discussed, in an online forum, two short stories illustrating dilemmas raised by the PBF sweater. Qualitative analysis of transcripts of the workshops and the forum identified patterns of moral argumentation in the reasoning processes by which participants challenge the PBF sweater's legitimacy: (1) when a shift in purpose occurs – from therapeutic to enhancement – and (2) when it engenders a shift in the user's sense of self – from an autonomous self to a socially coerced individual. These findings add nuance to current knowledge on public perceptions of cognitive and behavioural enhancement, providing insight into the ways that people conceive of the tension between autonomy and social coercion.

Human enhancement and public health

Human enhancement refers to the use of health products, medical procedures or technologies by healthy individuals to improve an attribute or ability (Evans-Brown, McVeigh, Perkins, & Bellis, 2012). In its *Health futures* horizon scanning report, the United Kingdom North West Public Health Observatory described enhancement practices as an 'emerging threat to health' (Evans-Brown et al., 2012, p. 16). Public health concerns include not only physiological, social and psychological harms, but also the more or less subtle moral changes that unfold over time and which render the use of certain enhancement technologies less reprehensible, i.e. normalized. In the past decades, ethics scholars have indeed called on public health practitioners and researchers to pay greater attention to the illicit and/or non-therapeutic use of pharmaceuticals by teenagers and young adults who wish to improve their cognitive functions, mood or social behaviours (Bell, Partridge, Lucke, & Hall, 2013; Lucke & Partridge, 2013; Outram & Racine, 2011; Racine, Waldman, Rosenberg, & Illes, 2010). In a similar vein, several wearable devices that 'collect data on one's bodily functions and everyday activities' (Lupton, 2013, p. 394) are now marketed directly to consumers in order to support or encourage a similar form of 'self-betterment' (Millington, 2016). The ease with which a growing number of people access such technologies and the sociocultural value attributed to having a better body, increasing one's well-being or empowering oneself could have a powerful influence on collective behaviour.

Acknowledging the moral and social underpinnings of new technologies that value 'good health above many other aspects of life and features of one's identity' (Lupton, 2013, p. 397), the aim of this paper is to examine how members of the public ponder the legitimacy of cognitive and behavioural enhancement. Using a combination of prospective multimedia material (i.e. videos and short stories taking place in 2030–2040), we conducted four face-to-face deliberative workshops with participants who later joined other participants in an asynchronous online forum to discuss a fictional 'smart' sweater that provides users with psycho-bio-feedback (PBF). Considering its potential to help adolescents to learn about and improve their cognitive, emotional and social skills, participants were invited to make explicit the desirable and undesirable aspects of the PBF sweater.

We first clarify the theoretical premises of our study and its qualitative methodology. Then, drawing on Swierstra and Rip's (2007) moral argumentation framework, our findings clarify participants' reasoning processes. These findings bring nuance to current work on public perception of enhancement technologies, while providing new insights into the way non-experts conceive of autonomy and social coercion.

Moral and social accounts of cognitive and behavioural enhancement technologies

Current research on public perceptions of cognitive and behavioural enhancement is mostly focused on the use of pharmaceuticals, e.g. methylphenidate (Ritalin®), mixed amphetamine salts (Adderall®) and modafinil (Provigil®). It sheds light on perceived risks and benefits (Bell et al., 2013; Thoer & Robitaille, 2011), media portrayal (Partridge, Bell, Lucke, Yeates, & Hall, 2011; Racine et al., 2010) and peer attitudes (DeSantis, Noar, & Webb, 2010; Dijkstra & Schuijff, 2016) that affect the perceptions and behaviours of users and non-users (typically, students or young adults) and of stakeholders (i.e. parents, health care providers, physicians; Hotze, Shah, Anderson, & Wynia, 2011). This body of research exposes the many ethical concerns underlying the distribution, consumption and regulation of cognitive and behavioural enhancement products, including rather novel ethical issues such as the shifting boundaries around what constitutes an authentic self (i.e. the value of one's genuine efforts devoted to self-development) (Schelle, Faulmüller, Caviola, & Hewstone, 2014). Yet, the illicit nature of the behaviour, alongside the fact that the available evidence mostly refers to students, limits our understanding of the meaning that individuals and groups attribute to such enhancement practices.

Few empirical studies have examined how users perceive and use wearable technologies (e.g. goggles, wristbands, sports shoes, weight scales), which through sensors 'woven into clothing or laminated onto ultrathin skin interfaces', provide a range of biometric data such as 'blood glucose, body temperature, breathing rate, blood chemistry readings, body weight, blood pressure, heart rate, sleep patterns, cardiac output readings and even brain activity' (Lupton, 2013, p. 397). According to Millington (2016, p. 408), technologies that 'automatically (or passively) register data with little effort required from people themselves' embody a 'healthism imperative' by making the body knowable in new ways and engaging users into personalized health surveillance. For Lupton (2013, p. 400), because such devices provide objectified data 'regardless of how well an individual may actually feel', they deserve in-depth research and analysis.

The theoretical premises of this paper sit at the interface between ethics, public health and Science and Technology Studies (STS). As Blaxter (1997) underscores, the way that lay people think and talk about health and illness not only differs from experts' conceptual frameworks, but it is also embedded in broad moral and social accounts that draw on shared identities. Aiming to clarify how society and technology coevolve, STS emphasize the linkages between experts' and non-experts' understandings of what counts as scientific and technological progress, of the boundaries between orthodox and non-orthodox health practices, and of what makes public policies legitimate or not (Boenink, Swierstra, & Stemerding, 2010; Calnan, Montaner, & Horne, 2005; Swierstra & Rip, 2007). STS also bring to the fore the way 'non-humans' (e.g. technical entities, systems, artifacts, etc.) make certain moral and social arrange-ments more persistent than others (Rock, Degeling, & Blue, 2014). Within this perspective, Millington (2016, p. 414) argued in favour of a critical public health scholarship that addresses how new forms of interaction between humans and non-humans give rise to 'posthuman optimization', wherein connected technologies become active health promotion agents.

To contribute such new insights to public health research on human enhancement, this paper draws on an analytical framework that emphasizes public reasoning processes, that is, the moral and social accounts through which people decide whether or not cognitive and behavioural enhancement prac-tices are desirable. For Swierstra and Rip (2007, p. 5), four categories of argument underpin moral debates around emerging technologies: (1) *consequentialist* arguments emphasizing benefits and risks; (2) arguments about *principles, duties and rights* that reflect deeply felt duty-based moral convictions; (3) arguments using theories of *justice* to question the social distribution of risks and benefits; and (4) arguments from *virtue ethics* conceptualizing the *good life*, i.e. 'who we are' and 'what we want to be'. These categories are distinct but accommodate both arguments in favour of or against a new technol-ogy (see Supplementary material, Table 1). For instance, although people may disagree on whether fair access to a given technology can be safeguarded, they may use the same moral argument (justice). This analytical framework thus highlights not only what people think, but also their moral reasoning processes, thereby clarifying the basis for attitudes towards an innovation (Stemerding, Swierstra, & Boenink, 2010).

Study design

Our multimedia-based deliberative study took place in Quebec (Canada) and was designed following Boenink and colleagues, for whom prospective scenarios are 'historically informed speculations' describ-ing possible futures (2010, p. 6). In our broader study, participants discussed three fictional technologies, including the PBF sweater. For each technology, we created a video clip that was discussed in four face-to-face deliberative workshops and two scenarios that were discussed through an asynchronous online forum with additional participants. For a detailed explanation of the development process of the fictional technologies and their multimedia material see the full protocol (Lehoux et al., 2014).

Multiple recruitment tools and strategies were deployed in parallel to constitute a purposeful study sample (Marshall & Rossman, 2011), targeting more specifically young adults (18–25), adults (30–55) and people over 60 years old. From the pool of interested participants, four groups were assembled: one group of young adults, one group of adults, one group of people over 60 years old and one mixed group. Using diversification criteria such as occupational profiles and hobbies, our goal was to obtain sufficient homogeneity in socio-economic status to ensure that the exchanges were comfortable and lively, yet diversified. A total of 38 participants attended the workshops and were invited to participate in

Table 1. Participant characteristics.

		n	%
Age	18–29	9	20
	30–39	6	13
	40–49	3	7
	50–59	7	15
	60–69	17	37
	>70	4	8
Gender	Female	33	72
	Male	13	28
Education	High school	4	9
	Collegial	5	11
	University	37	80
Household income	<$20,000	4	9
	$20,000 to $39,999	9	19
	$40,000 to $59,999	17	37
	>$60,000	16	35

the online forum (6 declined). Those people not available for the workshops were invited to the forum, to which a total of 57 participants contributed. Table 1 summarizes participant demographic profiles for the 46 participants who completed our survey.

The workshops were facilitated by a professional moderator. The video describing the PBF sweater was shown and then each participant was asked to share two to three desirable and two to three undesirable features with the group. A discussion ensued focusing on ways to improve the PBF sweater. The online forum – which ran over a five-week period, starting after the last workshop – was hosted on a login/password-secured blog platform (WordPress®) and facilitated by the same moderator. Participants were invited to read the scenarios and respond to questions to start the online deliberations. Box 1 summarizes the PBF sweater scenarios.

Box 1. A summary of how the PBF sweater and scenarios were presented to the participants.

Fictional technology's video presentation

- A sweater made of smart textiles with embedded sensors that provides, through an electronic device, real-time feedback about the mental state and cognitive performance of the person wearing it.

- When used in conjunction with meditation techniques, the sweater has the potential to help adolescents to learn about, and improve their cognitive abilities and social behaviours.

- In the video clip, an expert explains how the sweater has been used by students with learning difficulties and reduced dropout rates.

2030 scenario

- The sweater is now widely used by teenagers and integrated in school curricula as a learning tool for all students.

- Some experts call for prudence, estimating that it may negatively interfere with the user's perception of reality and identity.

2040 scenario

- The sweater use is mandatory during exams and enables the school to identify students' potential career paths as well as the classes they should follow.

- A student defies the school system by taking an exam without the PBF. Even if he successfully passed the exam, the school considers the results to be null since the procedure was not respected.

- To his parents' and friends' dismay, the student chooses to abandon the use of the PBF sweater and his initial career orientation.

The qualitative analysis software Dedoose™ facilitated the coding of the workshop transcripts (4 × 3.5 h) and online forum comments (*n* = 355). Swierstra and Rip's categories were used to identify the reasoning processes underlying the participants' appraisals of the (un)desirability of the PBF sweater. Examining code co-occurrence, many perceived qualities of the PBF were based on consequentialist arguments whereas arguments from the good life mostly emphasized criticisms (see Supplementary material, Table 2). Fewer accounts relied on the other two categories and emphasized as many desirable as undesirable features of the technology. Applying a constant comparative strategy (Strauss & Corbin, 1998) to further explore these variations, we observed that participants' reasoning processes challenged the PBF sweater's legitimacy: (1) when a shift in *purpose* occurred (therapy vs. enhancement); and (2) when it engendered a shift in the *user's sense of self* (autonomous person vs. socially coerced individual). Below, our findings clarify and illustrate why and how these two shifts in legitimacy occur. Quotes were translated from French to English and pseudonyms are used throughout the text.

Debating the (Un)desirability of the PBF sweater

Shift in purpose: from a remedy for learning deficits to performance enhancement

The problem the PBF sweater was meant to address – dropping out of school – was largely considered worthy of attention by participants, but their views regarding the technology's capacity to actually solve the problem diverged. For instance, Penelope wondered whether its effects would be sustained over time:

> When I heard 'to support reintegration' I thought, well … wow! Why not? And train the mind … there are aspects I found appealing, there's a playful side to it, but will its effect last? That remains to be seen. (Penelope, Workshop 1)

Because he saw the PBF sweater 'as a solution to a medical problem', Malik was 'really in favor':

> Dropping out of school, learning problems, that's medical to some extent. There are people who have dysphasia, people who have concentration problems, who have problems with stress and there are solutions to these problems; medical solutions in some cases, which helps a lot. Because when your personal stress prevents you from succeeding, I mean … it's not just because you're not interested in school: there's a barrier, it doesn't work, and that product gives you a chance. (Malik, Workshop 3)

Such consequentialist arguments were in general positive, emphasizing the value participants attribute to a technology that can remedy learning deficits or difficulties in managing one's emotions. For Karine, the idea that meditation techniques would be used alongside the PBF sweater 'could be interesting from a therapeutic point of view' considering that 'there's no one else within us'. It could also help 'someone who has panic attacks' (Karine, Workshop 2). In fact, when sharing ideas about ways to improve the PBF sweater, participants easily envisaged other potential therapeutic purposes. Charles was inspired by technological developments he knew about, including the remote monitoring of astronauts' vital signs:

> It would be brilliant [to use the PBF sweater] in a hospital after heart surgery, when the sternum has been cut in half, and the person is coughing too hard, which may imply risk of tear [laughs]. If sensors like that could support monitoring and coaching, such as 'listen, the data tell us that you're not careful, you don't put your pillow on your chest when coughing' it could avoid plenty of stuff. (Charles, Workshop 4)

Behavioural issues were also seen as candidate applications. Mary thought the PBF sweater would be 'extraordinary' for people with compulsive disorders:

> How many spend beyond their line of credit? I know of someone who ripped off $35,000 from his parents, just like that, last week. This person has to be controlled, *really* controlled. She'll get another credit card elsewhere, and elsewhere, and elsewhere. How do banks get to know? There should be a chip or I don't know what, that detects … And addictions … alcohol, gambling, all that. It'd be amazing to help the person, not just to control, but to help this person. I'm against profiling, but … those concerned such as banks, should have the means to detect these types of people. (Mary, Workshop 1)

Although it conflicts with the principle of autonomy, using the PBF sweater to restrain one's behaviour was a worthy purpose for Mary. In her account, intervening against a person's will could serve this person's best interests by minimizing the consequences of the compulsive disorder. For Simon, who was in the same group as Mary, using the PBF sweater with school dropouts was not considered therapeutic and thus deemed undesirable. But in 'listening to everyone' in the group, the application that he could see was for 'bullying and suicide'. He assumed that the technology could predict its user's mental distress:

> Someone who gets bullied wears this garment, then a signal will be sent to the school right away: 'ok, look he or she is being intimidated, we know he's on his way to suicide, we'll provide close support … because there's a risk of suicide'. (Simon, Workshop 1)

The purpose of improving student performance, which was introduced in the online scenarios (see Box 1), was rejected by all participants. Such a shift in purpose made clearer where participants drew a line between legitimate and illegitimate use of the PBF sweater: 'to blindly approve the daily wearing of a sweater that'll help [students] know themselves better, to live better with others, to always do better in their studies, that's the margin that I won't cross' (Line, Forum 2030). Schools were seen as competitive environments, driven by the quest for 'excellence' where one sees 'all that you do' and pervaded by a 'pressure to perform' (Homer, Workshop 4). Arguments about individual rights were used to criticize such a context of use; the PBF sweater could become a 'prerequisite' and 'anyone who did not use the PBF would be discriminated' (Baptiste, Forum 2030). From a justice perspective, the technology would be valuable to remedy learning deficits that handicap *certain* students and should be only used by 'those in need (learning disorders, anxiety, lack of confidence, etc.)' and who 'struggle at school' (Malik, Forum 2030).

Participants disapproved of using the PBF sweater to increase student performance, but not necessarily of improving human capacities in general. Samuel, from a good life perspective, was 'in favour of improving our capabilities through technology' and unwilling to 'go back and live without what the Internet and its search engines provide our youth'. He nonetheless found the race for performance illogical: 'I agree with Baptiste. If this sweater can help everyone, then every student who wants to become a physician will wear it and then the weakest will again be just as weak by comparison' (Samuel, Forum 2030). Relying on a justice argument, Adele pointed out that the value of the PBF sweater should be considered in light of its ability to protect those worst-off:

> What if tomorrow future employers force employees to wear this garment to increase their performance and access their brain? The idea gives me chills. An innovation must answer the question of its relevance – what problem does it fix? – and also address its social utility, i.e. how will relationships between humans be improved, how are those most vulnerable better protected. (Adele, Forum 2030)

Martin echoed the view of several participants when he argued that other solutions were needed to tackle the problem raised by dropouts, which 'can be fixed very differently by using our resources and by being creative' (Martin, Workshop 3). Like other participants who relied on good life arguments, Clemence proposed to put 'the human factor at the centre of life', which 'seems absolutely necessary to enable teens to live harmoniously' (Clemence, Forum 2030). The ubiquity of the Internet and its array of connected devices were seen as detrimental to the formation of human bonds, especially in a generation who grew up surrounded by such electronic devices.

To summarize, while participants voiced different opinions regarding the desirability of the PBF sweater, their reasoning processes emphasized that it could be medically justified if its purpose were to remedy a learning deficit but unwarranted if it primarily served an imperative of performance.

Shift in sense of self: from user self-development to coercive social uniformity

A second shift in participant accounts emerged when examining how they envisaged the nature of the PBF sweater's impact on its users. In contrast to medical technologies that address the physical dimension of diseases, the PBF sweater can shape the user's mind and behaviour. Hence, participants queried whether it would support self-development or coerce individuals into social uniformity.

Good life arguments stressed that the PBF sweater added an intermediary between one's feelings and one's inherent capacity to grasp such feelings, thereby reinforcing a hyper-rational sense of self. Both Jacques and Martin criticized this interference:

This product really has the quality ... the qualities of his defects actually. It's interesting to see the data it can give us access to, and on the other hand, it puts an interface between our feelings, our mental, physical state, etc. and our capacity to feel ... having to read in a Cartesian way, rationally on a screen, with schematized data versus just [asking myself] how I feel? (Jacques, Workshop 3)

It's a technology that prevents us from feeling ourselves, to be introspective, to take a moment to think about who we are, what we do, why we do it. We'll have beautiful indicators on a chart. And currently there are technologies like Fitbit that exist and which prevent people from realizing that when they run, they actually have pleasure while running. Rather, they have stats about their running. It disgusts me frankly! [laughs]. (Martin, Workshop 3)

Wondering 'who decides these social imperatives', Martin described the PBF sweater as 'a great social indoctrination method that should be used in all dictatorial societies of the world! [laughs]' (Workshop 3). Interestingly, Magalie drew on her previous experience as a teacher to make the counterpoint that the ability to develop oneself does require, at times, an external support and may entail a form of conditioning.

Because often the motivation must come from outside before a personal empowerment may begin. And the learning process about oneself is quite extraordinary ... the other merit I find is that it's a voluntary choice for conditioning. A person who wants to quit smoking or change his behaviour often needs this contribution, this external support ... In that sense, yes, it's a voluntary choice for conditioning. And I find it extraordinary. (Magalie, Workshop 3)

Magalie's argument reframes the basis upon which the principle of autonomy may be understood when it comes to a technology of the mind: may one freely choose to abandon his or her personal will? While participants appreciated the 'know thyself' approach (Clemence, Forum 2030) underlying the PBF sweater, many argued in favour of embedding its use within a set of coordinated services wherein adolescents are closely monitored and supported by professionals. This deontological view was supported by consequentialist arguments according to which the cost to society of a PBF sweater-centred professionalized programme could be offset 'by the savings generated by lower delinquency rates, social mischief and an increase in the employment rate and contribution to social and civic life' (Patricia, Forum 2040). A similar line of reasoning led Laura to stress that 'prevention is a must at an early age', but 'there'll always be dropouts who slip through the cracks of the school system'. Those teens for whom 'it's more difficult' to develop self-confidence, self-esteem and self-image 'need guidance, supervision and specialized help' (Laura, Forum 2030).

While participants valued a professional approach to self-development wherein the technology is used 'to develop knowledge about oneself' (Patricia, Forum 2040), they considered the many ways in which it could also threaten one's sense of self. Because 'there's a form of control in that sweater', Penelope wondered whether the teen would be 'comfortable, thinking one is trying to control me, trying to control my mind?' (Workshop 1). The feedback produced by the PBF sweater could generate adverse effects – 'I've got that sweater, it's in the red all the time and I'm good for nothing...' (Martin, Workshop 3) – and also threaten one's privacy:

Lea: I think it can traumatize the teenager.

Moderator: It might traumatize? Explanation...

Lea: Yes, when he feels controlled, 100%, as if someone is naked in front of everyone. It means he has no intimacy. It's ... I think it can traumatize the adolescent because at that age everyone has his own things and wants to keep his things personal. If everyone knows my weaknesses ... all my things in front of you...I think he will lose confidence in himself. (Lea, Workshop 4)

Participants queried whether the PBF sweater would *deprive* its users of cognitive and behavioural abilities; for instance, by inducing laziness it could reduce the 'learning capacity of the human being' (Baptiste, Forum 2030). For Gisele, the 'brain must make the effort to execute what is asked of it, otherwise it atrophies'. This is why when she was young, the use of the calculator 'was forbidden for simple multiplications and divisions' (Gisele, Forum 2030). From a good life standpoint, a technology that 'normalizes a neutral state' of mind and 'appeases everyone, whatever happens' may be 'downright dangerous' (Adele, Forum 2030). Line feared 'a generation of teens all alike, all calm, all dependent on a garment to feel good about themselves, just as they are sometimes when they consume medications or various drugs' (Forum 2030). The capacity to experience and handle social conflicts should be preserved: 'there are times when one must feel scandalized, refuse injustice, react' (Adele, Forum 2030). Similarly, Line underscored the importance of forging one's own personality and being able to challenge certain social values:

> Adolescence is a period where the values instilled are being questioned, and teens need this transitional period to find out who they really are and what they want to become. They need to be confronted with other values and different worldviews to find those that most resemble them. Of course, we all hope that these clashes happen in a non-violent manner, but sometimes one has to raise his voice, raise his arm straight to signify a disagreement. (Forum 2030)

To summarize, the fact that the PBF sweater could shape the mind and behaviour of its users led participants to ponder the ways in which it could interfere with sense of self. They appreciated the possibility of supporting a professionalized form of self-development if it fostered personal autonomy, but feared a world where everyone would be socially coerced into similar, behaviourally acceptable selves.

Discussion

We began this paper by underscoring the importance of understanding how different publics perceive human enhancement technologies since both experts' and non-experts' reasoning processes shape collective health practices (Dijkstra & Schuijff, 2016). After observing wide variation in physicians' willingness to prescribe both illicit and licit enhancement interventions (e.g. to suppress appetite, augment breast size, stimulate growth), Hotze and colleagues (2011, p. 11) concluded that 'an individual seeking an enhancement might be able to "doctor shop" to find a physician willing to prescribe almost any desired enhancement' be it pharmaceutical or technological.

Hence, in line with the call for empirical research on the ethical and technological dimensions of public health interventions (Green, 2014), our study examined the moral and social accounts through which members of the public considered the legitimacy of a fictional enhancement technology. Our participants' reasoning processes emphasized: (1) the PBF sweater's purpose, which could be considered medically justified if it remedied a learning deficit but unwarranted if it primarily served an imperative of performance; and (2) its impact on the user's sense of self, which could be desirable if it supported self-development but undesirable if it invalidated personal features by imposing social uniformity. By clarifying why and how these two shifts in legitimacy occur, our findings bring nuance to current work on public perception of enhancement technologies, while providing new insights into the way non-experts conceive of autonomy and social coercion.

First, our findings show that the legitimacy of the PBF sweater was not addressed in a vacuum: participants probed why, in what context and by whom it would be used. While they sometimes came to different conclusions, these intertwined considerations underpinned their overall judgment regarding whether or not it should be used. These findings lend support to Forlini and Racine's observation that it is important to examine the *circumstances* surrounding the use of enhancers (2012, p. 622). Using the PBF sweater to assess students' mental capacities and social skills, and to redirect their career paths, caused dismay; but the purpose of remedying learning deficits was seen as desirable. This is compatible with survey findings from Calnan and colleagues (2005) on public attitudes towards genetic technologies which revealed considerable 'ambivalence about human cloning and gene therapy to slow the ageing process but considerable support for genetic tests and stem cell therapy for the treatment of specific disorders'. In other words, 'treating or detecting diseases was valued but general interventions that aim to change "natural" processes were less acceptable' (2005, p. 1946). Drawing on a similar argument, Hotze and colleagues (2011, p. 11) explain physicians' frequent 'yes, but with reservations' survey responses: they 'might be willing to prescribe enhancement-type interventions only in limited circumstances, when those interventions might seem more like therapies'. Because our analytical framework made moral argumentation patterns more explicit, our findings clarify how consequentialist arguments highlighted the desirable features of the PBF sweater, i.e. its therapeutic virtues, whereas good life arguments underscored what made it undesirable, i.e. the social quest for performance. Participants thus expressed arguments that go beyond a clinical viewpoint, and moral nuances that contrast 'with the often strong and clear-cut pro and con positions encountered in the bioethics literature' (Forlini & Racine, 2012, p. 620). Overall, our study shows that members of the public do not reason according to mutually exclusive moral frameworks to make sense of why, in what context and for whom enhancement may be legitimate.

Second, our findings provide insight into the way people conceive of the tension between autonomy and social coercion. When pondering how the PBF sweater could interfere with sense of self, participants found desirable the idea of fostering a form of self-development that reinforces one's personal autonomy, but undesirable the idea of socially coercing individuals into similar selves. While there is a strong consensus around the importance of deciding autonomously, Thoer and Robitaille (2011) underscore that the use of enhancers cannot be conceptualized as the result of an individual decision or action; the students and young adults they interviewed obtained a prescription for, bought or exchanged drugs such as Ritalin® and Adderall® from friends, peers, parents or colleagues. In addition, they used these drugs as a form of coping strategy for dealing with work or school environments they considered too demanding and stressful. Public health scholars already know the importance of distinguishing between 'what is held to affect the health of society in general' and 'what is perceived as influential in one's own life' (Blaxter, 1997, p. 755). Yet, our findings suggest that the key issue at play is whether individuals can *still* be conceptualized as autonomous when one considers the broader socialized system of values in which they evolve, and where actively and successfully managing one's life represents a 'social injunction' (Thoer & Robitaille, 2011). While healthism reinforces a rational form of personal responsibility towards one's health, the 'pursuit of self-betterment' and self-optimization that underlies wearable technologies implies that responsibility is being partly delegated to 'sophisticated non-human devices' (Millington, 2016, p. 413). Our findings suggest that such devices may be considered, under certain conditions, therapeutic and thus legitimate. But when such devices are understood as shaping users into similar selves, members of the public are likely to resist their spread.

Study strengths and limitations

Our findings should be interpreted in light of our study's goals and limitations. Our sample was comprised of educated individuals, and more women than men agreed to participate; this type of sample is often found in public involvement studies (Street, Duszynski, Krawczyk, & Braunack-Mayer, 2014). Nonetheless, our study went beyond surveying student attitudes; we recruited participants aged from 19 to 72 year-old (33% were below 40 and 45% over 60). While individual interviews provide more space for participants to describe their views, our online component offered time and intimacy for participants to think about the scenarios before commenting (for a detailed assessment of the respective strengths and limitations of the multimedia components and of the two deliberative environments, see Lehoux, Jimenez-Pernett, Miller, & Williams-Jones, 2016). Our analytical framework was particularly relevant to our research goal and we reached empirical saturation around the two key themes described in this paper. While the framework did not exhaust all the empirical material (for instance, personal data privacy), it nevertheless increased the credibility of our analyses as well as its auditability (Marshall & Rossman, 2011). The transferability of our findings is limited to populations similar in terms of socio-economic and demographic composition, expectations towards publicly funded health systems and citizen engagement tradition. Overall, the key strengths of our study lie in the diversity of the participants we recruited, the use of videos and scenarios, the complementarity provided by two types of deliberative environment and the auditability of our analytical strategies.

Further research and concluding remarks

The emergence of cognitive and behavioural enhancement technologies calls for the development of new approaches to understand and tackle its implications for public health (Evans-Brown et al., 2012; Lupton, 2013). Most physicians surveyed by Hotze and colleagues believed that enhancement interventions that may 'produce discrete competitive life advantages' 'should be "allowed" (i.e. permitted, but not covered by insurance) but not "promoted" (i.e. covered by basic insurance plans)' (2011, p. 8). For these authors, 'to assert that "everyone should have equal access" to legal enhancement interventions, but that "they should not be covered by insurance"' entails a contradiction. Hence, further research should examine the public health underpinnings of a consequentialist appraisal of the benefits and risks of enhancement, which may indirectly reinforce its legitimacy: as long as *some* therapeutic benefits may be obtained in *some* individuals, enhancement is likely to be seen as morally acceptable. Yet, from a societal standpoint, arguments from a good life ethics would rather seek to clarify its 'moral praiseworthiness', i.e. is this a moral ideal to be actively supported? (Forlini & Racine, 2012, p. 621).

From a STS perspective, moral frameworks and new technological possibilities influence each other, giving rise to social and moral accounts that vary across space and time (Stemerding et al., 2010). By establishing linkages between the scholarly concerns of ethics, public health and STS, our study provides new insights into the way members of the public conceive of cognitive and behavioural enhancement and of the tension between autonomy and social coercion. The PBF sweater's legitimacy was challenged when a shift in purpose occurred – from therapeutic to enhancement – and when it engendered a shift in sense of self – from an autonomous self to a socially coerced individual. Because technological change affects public health research and practice in many different ways, STS-oriented studies (Rock et al., 2014) like ours are important to help understand the broader social and economic forces that shape the use of new technologies by opening up the inquiry to the human and non-human entities that 'inter-relate to produce and reproduce health and illness' (Green, 2014, p. 251).

Author's contributions

All authors revised the content of the manuscript and have approved the final version. PL is the principal investigator of the study; she is accountable for all aspects of the work, including the original idea behind the study and its development. BWJ, DG and SP have criticized earlier versions of the manuscript and contributed to the data analysis strategy, to the interpretation of the findings and to key conceptual and methodological decisions.

Competing interests

The authors declare that they have no competing interests.

Research ethics

The Health Research Ethics Committee of the University of Montreal approved the study and all participants provided informed consent.

Acknowledgements

This paper greatly benefitted from the constructivism criticisms of the Editor and two anonymous reviewers. A special thanks goes to Marianne Boenink whose work inspired this study. We would like to thank the study participants who generously contributed to our four workshops and online forum. Fiona A. Miller, Philippe Gauthier and Jennifer R. Fishman contributed to the broader study from which this paper stems by critically appraising preliminary versions of the research proposal before submission to the Canadian Institutes of Health Research (CIHR). Members of our research team – Myriam Hivon, Patrick Vachon, Geneviève Daudelin, Loes Knaapen, Olivier-Demers Payette and Jean Gagnon Doré – accomplished key tasks and shared insightful comments throughout the study. We also acknowledge the contribution of our Expert Committee members: Antoine Boivin, Amélie Doussau, Ghislaine Cleret de Langavant, Philippe Laporte, Lucie Nadeau, Nina Ndiaye, Vardit Ravitsky and Michel Venne.

Funding

This work was supported by the Canadian Institutes of Health Research [grant number CIHR; #MOP-119517]. P. Lehoux holds the University of Montreal Research Chair on Responsible Innovation in Health (2015–2018). Our research group infrastructure is supported by the *Fonds de la recherche du Québec-Santé* (FRQ-S). The study was approved by the Health Research Ethics Committee of the University of Montreal.

References

Bell, S., Partridge, B., Lucke, J., & Hall, W. (2013). Australian University students' attitudes towards the acceptability and regulation of pharmaceuticals to improve academic performance. *Neuroethics, 6*, 197–205.

Blaxter, M. (1997). Whose fault is it? People's own conceptions of the reasons for health inequalities. *Social Science & Medicine, 44*, 747–756.

Boenink, M., Swierstra, T., & Stemerding, D. (2010). Anticipating the interaction between technology and morality: A scenario study of experimenting with humans in bionanotechnology. *Studies in Ethics, Law, and Technology, 4*, 1941–6008.

Calnan, M., Montaner, D., & Horne, R. (2005). How acceptable are innovative health-care technologies? A survey of public beliefs and attitudes in England and Wales. *Social Science & Medicine, 60*, 1937–1948.

DeSantis, A., Noar, S. M., & Webb, E. M. (2010). Speeding through the frat house: A qualitative exploration of nonmedical ADHD stimulant use in fraternities. *Journal of Drug Education, 40*, 157–171.

Dijkstra, A. M., & Schuijff, M. (2016). Public opinions about human enhancement can enhance the expert-only debate: A review study. *Public Understanding of Science, 25*, 588–602.

Evans-Brown, M., McVeigh, J., Perkins, C., & Bellis, M. A. (2012). *Human enhancement drugs: The emerging challenges to public health*. Liverpool: North West Public Health Observatory.

Forlini, C., & Racine, E. (2012). Stakeholder perspectives and reactions to "academic" cognitive enhancement: Unsuspected meaning of ambivalence and analogies. *Public Understanding of Science, 21*, 606–625.

Green, J. (2014). What kind of research does public health need? *Critical Public Health, 24*, 249–252.

Hotze, T. D., Shah, K., Anderson, E. E., & Wynia, M. K. (2011). "Doctor, would you prescribe a pill to help me … ?" A national survey of physicians on using medicine for human enhancement. *The American Journal of Bioethics, 11*, 3–13.

Lehoux, P., Gauthier, P., Williams-Jones, B., Miller, F. A., Fishman, J. J., Hivon, H., & Vachon, P. (2014). Examining the ethical and social issues of health technology design through the public appraisal of prospective scenarios: A study protocol describing a multimedia-based deliberative method. *Implementation Science, 9*, 81. doi: 10.1186/1748-5908-9-81

Lehoux, P., Jimenez-Pernett, J., Miller, F. A., & Williams-Jones, B. (2016). Assessment of a multimedia-based prospective method to support public deliberations on health technology design: Participant survey findings and qualitative insights. *BMC Health Services Research, 16*, 616. doi: 10.1186/s12913-016-1870-z

Lucke, J., & Partridge, B. (2013). Towards a smart population: A public health framework for cognitive enhancement. *Neuroethics, 6*, 419–427.

Lupton, D. (2013). Quantifying the body: Monitoring and measuring health in the age of mHealth technologies. *Critical Public Health, 23*, 393–403.

Marshall, C., & Rossman, G. B. (2011). *Designing qualitative research*. Thousand Oaks, CA: Sage.

Millington, B. (2016). 'Quantify the invisible': Notes toward a future of posture. *Critical Public Health, 26*, 405–417.

Outram, S. M., & Racine, E. (2011). Developing public health approaches to cognitive enhancement: An analysis of current reports. *Public Health Ethics, 4*, 93–105.

Partridge, B. J., Bell, S. K., Lucke, J. C., Yeates, S., & Hall, W. D. (2011). Smart drugs "as common as coffee": Media hype about neuroenhancement. *Plos One, 6*, e28416.

Racine, E., Waldman, S., Rosenberg, J., & Illes, J. (2010). Contemporary neuroscience in the media. *Social Science & Medicine, 71*, 725–733.

Rock, M. J., Degeling, C., & Blue, G. (2014). Toward stronger theory in critical public health: Insights from debates surrounding posthumanism. *Critical Public Health, 24*, 337–348.

Schelle, K. J., Faulmüller, N., Caviola, L., & Hewstone, M. (2014). Attitudes toward pharmacological cognitive enhancement: A review. *Frontiers in Systems Neuroscience, 8*, 1–14.

Stemerding, D., Swierstra, T., & Boenink, M. (2010). Exploring the interaction between technology and morality in the field of genetic susceptibility testing: A scenario study. *Futures, 42*, 1133–1145.

Strauss, A., & Corbin, J. (1998). *Basics of qualitative research: Techniques and procedures for developing grounded theory*. Thousand Oaks, CA: Sage.

Street, J., Duszynski, K., Krawczyk, S., & Braunack-Mayer, A. (2014). The use of citizens' juries in health policy decision-making: A systematic review. *Social Science & Medicine, 109*, 1–9.

Swierstra, T., & Rip, A. (2007). Nano-ethics as NEST-ethics: Patterns of moral argumentation about new and emerging science and technology. *NanoEthics, 1*, 3–20.

Thoer, C., & Robitaille, M. (2011). Utiliser des médicaments stimulants pour améliorer sa performance: usages et discours de jeunes adultes québécois [Using stimulant drugs to improve one's performance: uses and discourses of young adults in Quebec]. *Drogues, santé et société, 10*, 143–183.

COMMENTARY

Pigs in public health

Mette N. Svendsen

ABSTRACT
Animals are rare topics in public health science texts and speech despite the fact that animal bodies and lives are woven into the health of human populations, and vice versa. Years of ethnographic and documentary research – following pigs and their humans in and out of biomedical research – made me mindful and watchful of the porous passages between animal and human bodies and environments that do not confine themselves to 'national health programs' directed towards a specific (human) population. These unrecognized species encounters and relationships, which exceed the conventional framework of public health, made me re-evaluate both what 'public' and what 'health' means in public health. In this commentary I provide a short personal account of that intellectual journey. I argue that entanglements between species make it urgent that public health scholars investigate the moral, socio-economic, material, and bacterial passages between humans and animals that constitute the various publics of public health and profoundly shape the health of human and animal populations in a globalized world.

'It is just a pig, why bother?' my friend asks with a hint of annoyance in her voice. We are chatting over a cup of coffee in the fall of 2010 and I have just told her about my ethnographic fieldwork in an animal facility at the University of Copenhagen and in the neonatal intensive care unit (NICU) at the university hospital nearby. In the first site, I follow experiments on hyper-sensitive and highly compromised premature piglets in incubators; experiments that aim at optimizing nutrition for infants at risk of the serious gut disease necrotizing enterocolitis (NEC). In the second site, I follow clinical decision-making around infants at the very fringes of life, some of them born as early as gestation week 23. They are the infants whose health the animal experiments seek to improve. The 'just a pig' comment echoes conversations with my colleagues in public health. Introducing them to my research into how developments in medical technology are pushing the limits of life across species and raising pressing concerns about human lives, in particular, they all immediately understood my interest in clinical decision-making and questions about withdrawal or continuation of treatment for premature infants in neonatology. Just a few introductory sentences about this field immediately provoked outbursts about the urgency of my study, questions about the disability risks of being born prematurely, emphatic responses to the parents' precarious situation, and caring comments about how challenging it must be for me personally to be part of this field facing the ethical challenges and sufferings of families on a daily basis. On the contrary, the pig component of the research, which I also often happened to talk about in a lighthearted tone of voice, made us smile or laugh. The fact that I approached the constellation of 'just pigs' in incubators with the same set of questions that I approached the constellation of infants in incubators was hilarious. What did a social scientist do in an animal facility? Was it the case that against all their expectations I happened to be an animal rights person or a vegetarian? Relief entered my colleagues' faces when they learned that was not the case. Thus, while the research questions I raised in the NICU were recognizable to people and had great support, the same questions raised in relation to pigs questioned my professional and personal identity. The notion of the pig as simply a resource for human players, as just meat, penetrated every conversation with friends in my house and with colleagues on campus.

In my public health department, the 'pig project' – that Lene Koch and I, and two graduate students, were engaged in – was often mentioned as an example of the broadness of the public health field and its many strange corners. I, too, shared this conception of 'our pigs' as remotely positioned from core areas of public health concerned with disease risks and their connection to life styles, genetics, socio-economic status, gender, national health policies, health care systems, and preventive interventions. However, moving between the NICU and the animal facility unravelling connections between these sites and the Danish welfare society, I not only began to view the pig differently, but came to see the pig as central to the field of public health. More profoundly, following pigs in and out of biomedical research made me re-evaluate my notions of both 'public' and 'health' in public health.

Unrecognized entanglements

During the ethnographic fieldwork that I – and later graduate student Laura E. Navne – conducted in the NICU, I only rarely spotted comments on the animal-based origin of the treatment used. Once, a physician in passing commented that he would put a vein from a calf into a child who was to undergo a heart operation. The clinicians did not inform the parents about this calf vein in the heart of their child. In the parents' stressful situation following premature birth and the shock of learning about their infant's complicated heart disease, a calf vein was an unimportant piece of information. Similarly, when infants were provided with the drug surfactant that is isolated from minced pig lungs, the clinicians did not consider the animal origin of this drug important and there was certainly no mentioning of the pig in conversations among the clinicians or with the parents.

In the animal facility, however, there was no way to escape the materiality of the pig. As the team gathered around the 300-kg anaesthetized pregnant sow, which had come into the animal facility from a piggery outside Copenhagen, the operation theatre smelled of the animal body heavily asleep in front of us. From its mouth and snout sounded a loud snoring; from the other end, urine splashed down on the floor. The associate professor in charge of the surgery instructed her students in how to cut through the skin. Everyone followed how one piglet after the other (20 in total) were taken out of the womb and handed from the professor to members of the research team. Soon afterwards, the piglets were moved to a separate room and placed in heated, individual, incubator-like cages. The piglets were divided into groups and through an oral tube provided with different forms of nutrition – e.g. human donor milk, bovine colostrum and ordinary formula – given with the same technology and at the same intervals as given to infants in the NICU. Through the following five days, the piglets were taken care of by the research team who attended to them constantly. On day five, the piglets were killed and their bodies turned into samples to be analysed in the laboratory with the aims of reaching new insights into severe paediatric diseases such as NEC, and of improving feeding regimes and rearing conditions in the critical neonatal period.

Although the researchers spent days and nights in the pig laboratory running these experiments and taking care of the piglets, when presenting their research to strangers they always began their narrative in the clinic despite the fact that they might have visited the NICU only once. The risk of NEC in premature infants and the need for a cure constituted the plot that carved out a central role for the researchers in alliance with the pig to improve public health. The infants – not the mother sow from the farm – were the central actors in the origin stories (Morgan, 2009) that the researchers told themselves and others about their research and the piglets in their care. In leaving out the sow and Danish pork production, their stories mirrored the absence of the animals in the clinic and the absence of animals in public announcements of medical breakthroughs that often labelled the laborious work with animals as simply 'animal based experiments'.

Through periods of participant observations in 2009 and 2011 (carried out by me) and in 2013 (carried out by graduate student Mie S. Dam) I came to know 'animal based experiments' as a social and material space. With inspiration from an expanding social science literature on human–animal relationships (Candea, 2010; Davies, 2012; Haraway, 2008; Kohn, 2007; Yates-Doerr, 2015) and the role of animals in the becoming of particular human publics (Franklin, 2007; Friese, 2014; Sharp, 2013), I followed the day-to-day practices of caring for and killing the piglets in the animal facility. During experimental weeks, it was paramount for the researchers that the animals became sick from the same deadly gut infections as infants in the NICU, yet it was also paramount that the piglets did not suffer unnecessarily and that they did not die (from other diseases) before the scheduled 'kill day' as this would prevent the researchers from observing how the animals responded to different forms of nutrition. To achieve this goal of keeping the piglets in life to the end of the experiment took much individual care within the otherwise highly standardized experiment. Constantly checking on the piglets, calling in an experienced colleague discussing whether to take out a little bit of air from one piglet's stomach or regulating the heat or the amount of food of another animal, the researchers did not merely approach the piglets as standardized biology, but as sentient individuals.

In this setting, the care performed to make the animals live on to the last day of the experiment played a constitutive role in the organization of the experimental practice and shaped the animal bodies and the findings that resulted from them (Friese, 2013). That is, the care work was not simply something 'extra' apart from the protocol. It was essential to running the studies (keeping the piglets alive) and in some cases it was also a way of bringing the piglets closer to the individualized care in the NICU. Hybrid human-animal identities emerged (Dam & Svendsen, in press). Thus, in one week a limp piglet was continuously named 'the loser' (Skidtmads), in another week, a weak piglet was named 'mousy' (musse), and usually during experiments the most thriving piglets would be called 'darling' (kælegris). Often, the researchers jokingly addressed the piglets as if they were their infants, for instance closing a feeding session by saying, 'goodnight my babies'. During some studies in 2013, the group researched the relationship between gut and brain and invented ways of measuring the piglets' cognitive development. To do so they needed a longer perspective than the five days that their usual model runs and initiated a set of studies lasting 26 days during which individual care was even more important. In one of these studies, one of the masters students provided each piglet with the name of a Nobel Prize winner such as Albert Einstein, Conrad Röntgen, and Andrew Huxley. The irony involved in all of these naming situations treated the piglets as persons in Marcel Mauss's sense of acting under a set of descriptions (Mauss, 1985). The names, together with the extensive log books documenting the health situation of each piglet during the study, momentarily made them into biographical lives spatially belonging in the 'household' of the research group, who had their offices on the floor above the pig laboratory (Svendsen, 2016; Svendsen & Koch, 2013).

This care work as well as the killing on the last day of the experiment opened the label 'animal based experiments' to me. In hearing about new treatment advancements or reading about old breakthroughs in neonatology such as the positive outcome of the combination of surfactant treatment with nCPAP (nasal continuous positive airflow pressure) in infants with moderate-to-severe respiratory distress (Verder et al., 1994), I now see these infant cohorts as standing on populations of pigs whose lungs constitute the crucial ingredient in surfactant, and on populations of newborn lambs (Ikegami, Jobe, & Glatz, 1981) and of rabbits (Robertson, Curstedt, Johansson, Jörnvall, & Kobayashi, 1990) on which the surfactant therapy was tested. That is, I have become tuned into how the human public is entangled with research animal biographies (Pihl, 2017), housing arrangements (Bjørkdahl & Druglitrø, 2016), and endless relationships to non-human actors – protocols, catheters, tubes, nutrition, knives, excel spreadsheets – which Science and Technology Studies have foregrounded and demonstrated as holding analytical potential (Latour & Woolgar, 1986; Law, 2002; Mol, 2002; see also Will this volume). Stepping into the animal facility made me consider the human, not as a natural point of origin for public health, but as an achievement that relied on 'unrecognized entanglements' with an 'underground common'

(Tsing, 2015, p. 274) of non-humans. In other words, I became aware of the public fiction (Mathews, 2011) of 'animal based experiments' and the many actors this fiction makes unknown (cf. Geissler, 2013). While there are good reasons for the doctors in the NICU not to inform parents about the animal connection in the treatment of their infants, to scholars in public health there are indeed very good reasons to investigate exactly this interface between human and non-human actors. Studying this interface provides a lens for understanding how a given 'public' in public health comes into being, and which exchanges with other forms of life it relies on. In this way 'derailing the human' (Rees, in press) creates an avenue into understanding the social genesis of public health.

Pigs and health

Although the researchers in the animal facility would always begin the story about their pig experiments in the NICU, my friend's comment, 'It is just a pig', hinted at an equally important origin story of their research. As the researchers told me many times, in Denmark we raise and kill close to 30 million pigs annually, more than four times the human population. Consequently, the use of pigs in biomedical laboratories not only reflects the great expertise on pig biology in Danish veterinary science, but also that treating the pig as a tool for human health grows out of a long Danish tradition for turning the pig body into welfare for humans.

With no extensive natural resources, the main assets of Denmark are its people and their farm animals, most significantly Danish pigs which since the nineteenth century have been an important economic resource for the nation. When Denmark became a world leader in the export of pork, especially bacon for the British market, the strong national economic dependence on this export meant that economic and foreign policy was sensitive to demands from the pork industry. Throughout the twentieth century, pig production has expanded and continued to provide a sizable income for the Danish state. Along with other income-generating export industries, pig production has contributed to public institutions such as hospitals and public health interventions.

In the last decades, the importance of pork production for the Danish welfare state has become increasingly contested in response to a debt-ridden agricultural sector, the pollution of Danish waters due to discharge of slurry, and, most recently, the increase and spread of the antibiotic-resistant methicillin-resistant staphylococcus aureus (MRSA) bacteria in Danish piggeries. The MRSA controversy pertains to the ways in which the widespread use of antibiotics in pig production puts human health at risk as the MRSA bacteria is transmitted from pigs to pig farmers and from them to other parts of the population. As an example, in the NICU in 2014 a few staff-members and infants were infected with MRSA. Although the relationship between 'environment' and 'health risks' is central to public health, livestock farming and zoonoses are rare topics in the curriculum of public health students at the University of Copenhagen unless they specialize in global health where humans and animals presumably always have closer relationships than in public health 'classic'. However, the political attention to the current stream of travelling microbes from animal farming to human health care reminds us to imagine bodies as 'permeable interfaces of active traffic' (Solomon, 2016, p. 5) and think in terms of porous passages between bodies and environments. The MRSA controversy profoundly reconfigured my sense of health in the realm of public health. Where at the beginning of my research I placed myself in a foregrounded human public whose health was shaped by (human) life styles, national health programmes, discourses, health care services, and genetics, I increasingly saw this 'public' as a small local island in a world inhabited by all kinds of species, technologies, policies, practices and economies suffusing the human public (Rock, Degeling, & Gwendolyn, 2014). This forced me to foreground the multi-species environments that suffuse it (see Solomon, 2016, p. 73), so that the pigs that at first sight seemed 'outside' of human public health ended up being located 'inside' the classic public health field of preventing disease and promoting health.

If populations of livestock piglets are brought into life in the laboratory as part of experiments aimed at improving nutrition for future human infants at the fringes of life, how, then, is the population of livestock pigs being fed in Denmark? This question is based in an interest in the above-mentioned permeable passages between environments and earthly inhabitants – what we may also think of as metabolic relations across species in a globalized world (Law & Mol, 2008). Despite the fact that Denmark is the most intensively cultivated country in the world (62% of Danish land is farmland), the cultivated fields in Denmark are not sufficient to feed close to 30 million pigs a year. Therefore, Denmark has a yearly import of 1.2 million tons of genetically modified soybeans from the Amazon (Bosselmann & Gylling, 2012). Thus, the landscape and lives involved in the local biology of the Danish pig and the local practices of upholding the pig as an economic resource for Denmark reach far beyond the Danish borders. In South America, the production of soy for the world food market has dramatically changed the landscape and the economy in the Amazon and created environmental concerns because of destruction of the high concentration of biodiversity in production zones. Add to this health problems and death among workers because of the extended use of pesticides, and socio-economic problems because of the increasing poverty among workers (Lapegna, 2016; Nepstad, Stickler, & Almeida, 2006; Steward, 2007) as big multinational firms dominate the soybean production and concentrate profits in a relatively small number of hands (de Sousa & Vieira, 2008, p. 238). Ethnography from the Amazon suggests that for the local populations the soybeans have increasing become 'killer beans' (Hetherington, 2013). The soy for Danish pigs is a microscopic share of all the South American soy produced for the world market and it is difficult to trace from which fields and corporations Danish pig farmers get their soy, yet the Danish import still demonstrates that what may *look like* a local nationally bounded health and welfare (pig) source in one part of the world, *actually* draws upon inequalities in welfare possibilities in a global world. What becomes a source of good health for one public (e.g. lean pork meat and improved nutrition for neonates 'based on animal experiments') is deeply entangled with the health and welfare of other beings – humans and non-humans – in other sectors of our society or other parts of the world.

The above reflections are in no way new to scholars in public health. As academics and citizens we are aware of both the socio-economic inequalities in a global world and the microbial passages between animals and humans that shape human and animal health, and thus are at the heart of the 'health' in public health. What is remarkable is the way in which my colleagues and I indulged in laughing about my pig study. In doing so we continued to perform the public fiction that the health of the public is solely about health behaviour, discourses, institutions and distributions of risks set within a bounded entity of a 'health care system' or a particular (human) population. My friend was right in directing my attention to the fact that 'it is just a pig'. By unravelling the 'just' and the 'pig' we may discover the moral, socio-economic, material, and bacterial passages that connect our island of public health to other species. The attentive reader may note that my way of derailing the human continues to bring me back to the human. Ultimately, my study is not about how pigs live their lives, but their relationship with humans and their role in human publics. Like most public health scholars, I take an interest in human populations. However, following pigs and humans between agriculture, experimental laboratory science, and clinical practice has taught me to stay aware of origin stories that embrace more than human collectivities. In other words, it is time to let our critical public health gaze inspect what is made unknown in delineating human populations and to take seriously the multiplicity of passages between bodies and environments in a global world. From that position we may ask anew how a public comes into being and how the health of this population is entangled with the lives of other populations, human as well as non-human.

Acknowledgements

Insights discussed in this commentary are gained from research supported by grants from the Danish Research Councils (*Life at the Margins* and *A Life Worth Living* (Sapere Aude) and from my participation in the research platform NEOMUNE. Thank you to Lene Koch, Mie. S. Dam, Iben M. Gjødsbøl, and Laura E. Navne for great companionship in bringing animals into public health and for very helpful advice on this commentary.

Disclosure statement

No potential conflict of interest was reported by the author.

Funding

This research was supported by the Danish Research Councils [grant number 0602-00854B], [grant number 12-133657].

References

Bjørkdahl, K., & Druglitrø, T. (2016). *Animal housing and human-animal relations: Politics, practices and infrastructures*. London: Routledge.

Bosselmann, A. S., & Gylling, M. (2012). *Danmarks rolle i de globale værdikæder for konventionel og certificeret soja og palmeolie* [The role of Denmark in the global value chain for conventional and certified soy and palm oil]. Copenhagen: FOI Udredning, Department of Food and Resource Economics, Copenhagen University.

Candea, M. (2010). "I fell in love with Carlos the meerkat": Engagement and detachment in human–animal relations. *American Ethnologist, 37*, 241–258.

Dam, M. S., & Svendsen, M. N. (in press). Treating pigs: Balancing standardisation and individual treatments in translational neonatology research. *Biosocieties*.

Davies, G. (2012). What is a humanized mouse? Remaking the species and spaces of translational medicine. *Body and Society, 18*, 126–155.

de Sousa, I. F. S., & Vieira, R. C. M. T. (2008). Soy beans and soy foods in Brazil with notes on Argentina. In C. Du Bois, C.-B. Tan, & S. Mintz (Eds.), *The world of soy* (pp. 234–256). Urbana and Chicago, IL: University of Illinois Press.

Franklin, S. (2007). *Dolly mixtures*. Durham, NC: Duke University Press.

Friese, C. (2013). Realizing potential in translational medicine. *Current Anthropology, 54*(Suppl. 7), 129–138.

Friese, C. (2014). *Cloning wildlife: Zoos, captivity, and the future of endangered animals*. New York: New York University Press.

Geissler, P. W. (2013). Public secrets in public health: Knowing not to know while making scientific knowledge. *American Ethnologist, 40*, 13–34.

Haraway, D. J. (2008). *When species meet*. Minneapolis: University of Minnesota Press.

Hetherington, K. (2013). Beans before the law: Knowledge practices, responsibility, and the Paraguayan soy boom. *Cultural Anthropology, 28*, 65–85.

Ikegami, M., Jobe, A., & Glatz, T. (1981). Surface activity following surfactant treatment in premature lambs. *Journal of Applied Physiology: Respiratory, Environmental and Exercise Physiology, 51*, 306–312.

Kohn, E. (2007). How dogs dream: Amazonian natures and the politics of transspecies engagement. *American Ethnologist, 34*, 3–24.

Lapegna, P. (2016). *Soybeans and power*. New York, NY: Oxford University Press.

Latour, B., & Woolgar, S. (1986). *Laboratory life: The construction of scientific facts*. Princeton, NJ: Princeton University Press.

Law, J. (2002). *Aircraft stories*. Durham, NC: Duke University Press.

Law, J., & Mol, A. (2008). Globalisation in practice: On the politics of boiling pigswill. *Geoforum, 39*, 133–143.

Mathews, A. (2011). *Instituting nature*. Cambridge, MA: MIT Press.

Mauss, M. (1985). A category of the human mind: The notion of person; the notion of self. In M. Carrithers, S. Collins, & S. Lukes (Eds.), *The category of the person: Anthropology, philosophy, history* (pp. 1–25). Cambridge: Cambridge University Press (First published 1938).

Mol, A. (2002). *The body multiple*. Durham, NC: Duke University Press.

Morgan, L. (2009). *Icons of life*. Berkeley: University of California Press.

Nepstad, D. C., Stickler, C. M., & Almeida, O. T. (2006). Globalization of the Amazon soy and beef industries: Opportunities for conservation. *Conservation Biology, 20*, 1595–1603.

Pihl, V. (2017). Making pig research biographies: Names and numbers. In K. Asdal, T. Druglitrø, & S. Hinchliffe (Eds.), *The more-than-human-condition* (pp. 48–65). London: Routledge.

Rees, T. (in press). *After ethnos. Sketches of a deanthropologized anthropology*. Durham, NC: Duke University Press.

Robertson, B., Curstedt, T., Johansson, J., Jörnvall, H., & Kobayashi, T. (1990). Structural and functional characterization of porcine surfactant isolated from liquid-gel chromatography. *Basic Research on Lung Surfactant, 25*, 237–246.

Rock, M. J., Degeling, C., & Gwendolyn, B. (2014). Toward stronger theory in critical public health: Insights from debates surrounding posthumanism. *Critical Public Health, 24*, 337–348.

Sharp, L. A. (2013). *Transplant imaginary*. Berkeley: University of California Press.

Solomon, H. (2016). *Metabolic living*. Durham, NC: Duke University Press.

Steward, C. (2007). From colonization to "Environmental Soy": A case study of environmental and socio-economic valuation in the Amazon soy frontier. *Agriculture and Human Values, 24*, 107–122.

Svendsen, M. N. (2016). The spatial arrangements of making research piglets into resources for translational medicine. In K. Bjørkdahl & T. Druglitrø (Eds.), *Animal housing and human-animals relations: Politics, practices and infrastructures* (pp. 185–198). London: Routledge.

Svendsen, M. N., & Koch, L. (2013). Potentializing the research piglet in experimental neonatal research. *Current Anthropology, 54*(Suppl. 7), 118–128.

Tsing, A. (2015). *The mushroom at the end of the world*. Princeton, NJ: Princeton University Press.

Verder, H., Robertson, B., Greisen, G., Ebbesen, F., Albertsen, P., Lundstrøm, K., & Jacobsen, T. (1994). Surfactant therapy and nasal continuous positive airway pressure for newborns with respiratory distress syndrome. *New England Journal of Medicine, 331*, 1051–1055.

Will, C. (2017). On difference and doubt as tools for critical engagement with public health. *Critical Public Health*. doi: 10.1080/09581596.2016.1239815

Yates-Doerr, E. (2015). Does meat come from animals? A multispecies approach to classification and belonging in highland Guatemala. *American Ethnologist, 42*, 309–323.

Index

Milton Keynes UK
Ingram Content Group UK Ltd.
UKHW051855071024
449327UK00025B/1970